"The body has a privileged status in contemporary thinking, but it typically marks the point at which thinking stops and brute material reality is asserted. Sarah Meehan O'Callaghan's stunning *Psychoanalysing Mind-Body Narratives through Beckett and Artaud* marks a radical break from this unfortunate tendency. Through the narratives of Beckett and Artaud, O'Callaghan finds how the body appears not as a limit that thought cannot surpass but as a point of impossibility within thought. Through her approach, she discovers a compelling new way of conceiving the mind-body problem, as this relationship becomes the expression of subjectivity itself. A revolutionary work for a world in which we are losing touch with the body as its priority becomes more vehemently asserted."

**Professor Todd McGowan**, *University of Vermont, USA*

"While providing original and insightful analyses of key Beckett and Artaud theatre works, this book makes a vital contribution to the intersection of psychoanalysis and embodiment studies. It draws on the Lacanian Real to argue that that the body is fundamentally unknowable, but that cultural narratives or visual fantasies of the ideal, able and productive body seek to elide this foundational gap in our knowledge and the trauma it produces. Sarah Meehan O'Callaghan argues that, in very different ways, the theatre of these two playwrights, in theory as well as practice in Artaud's case, work on the spectator to dismantle the normative perceptual, linguistic and representational structures that conceal the ontological trauma of embodiment. This trauma is part of the human condition of both having and being a body but is most acutely experienced by those who are marginalised through illness, age or disability. Through her readings of Beckett and Artaud's theatre, the author powerfully challenges those narratives and images of normative embodiment in culture, aesthetics and psychoanalysis. Beautifully written, this is a carefully argued and accessible account of the relevance of Lacanian theory to the fact that 'when it comes to our relation to the body, we are not masters in our own homes'."

**Professor Anna McMullan**, *Professor in Theatre and Director of Research for Film, Theatre and Television, University of Reading, UK*

# Psychoanalysing Mind–Body Narratives through Beckett and Artaud

This book provides an epistemology of the body as it relates to subjectivity through an analysis of selected works of Antonin Artaud and Samuel Beckett. Presented in three parts, the book explores a fundamental premise: that there is a traumatic and alienating dimension to embodiment that resists expression within representational systems and is core to the being of any subject.

In Part One, The Epistemology of the Body, Meehan O'Callaghan approaches a theory of the body as traumatic by framing it as a question, a gap in knowledge, through the lens of psychoanalysis and theatre studies. Part Two, The Body of Drama, is devoted to a study of the body in the works of Beckett and Artaud from the perspective of psychoanalysis. Part Three, The Body Between Being and Non-Being, provides a deeper exploration of how the interrogation of the body opens onto a question of being and uses the insights gained from the dialectical encounter of psychoanalysis with the specific works of Beckett and Artaud to apply them to contemporary and scholarly issues of the body.

*Psychoanalysing Mind–Body Narratives through Beckett and Artaud* will be essential reading for psychoanalysts in practice and in training, and for academics and scholars of Lacanian studies, psychoanalytic studies, the body, disability studies, and literary and theatre studies.

**Sarah Meehan O'Callaghan** is an independent scholar, editor, and writer. She has published numerous articles and book chapters in the field of Lacanian psychoanalysis, covering topics such as sexuality, disability, ethics, and the body. She is the founder of Visionediting, a business devoted to editing and writing.

## The Lines of the Symbolic in Psychoanalysis Series

Series Editor: Ian Parker, Manchester Psychoanalytic Matrix

Psychoanalytic clinical and theoretical work is always embedded in specific linguistic and cultural contexts and carries their traces, traces which this series attends to in its focus on multiple contradictory and antagonistic 'lines of the Symbolic'. This series takes its cue from Lacan's psychoanalytic work on three registers of human experience, the Symbolic, the Imaginary and the Real, and employs this distinctive understanding of cultural, communication and embodiment to link with other traditions of cultural, clinical and theoretical practice beyond the Lacanian symbolic universe. The Lines of the Symbolic in Psychoanalysis Series provides a reflexive reworking of theoretical and practical issues, translating psychoanalytic writing from different contexts, grounding that work in the specific histories and politics that provide the conditions of possibility for its descriptions and interventions to function. The series makes connections between different cultural and disciplinary sites in which psychoanalysis operates, questioning the idea that there could be one single correct reading and application of Lacan. Its authors trace their own path, their own line through the Symbolic, situating psychoanalysis in relation to debates which intersect with Lacanian work, explicating it, extending it and challenging it.

**Queer Psychoanalysis: Minor Clinic and Deconstruction of Gender**
*Fabrice Bourlez*

**A Contemporary Return to the Lacanian Mirror: You Are That**
*Sergio J. Aguilar Alcalá*

**Writings for a Liberation Psychoanalysis: Politicizing the Unconscious from the Core of a Crumbling Empire**
*Robert K. Beshara*

**Psychoanalysing Mind–Body Narratives Through Beckett and Artaud: The Trauma of the Body**
*Sarah Meehan O'Callaghan*

For more information about the series, please visit: https://www.routledge.com/The-Lines-of-the-Symbolic-in-Psychoanalysis-Series/book-series/KARNLOS

# Psychoanalysing Mind–Body Narratives through Beckett and Artaud

## The Trauma of the Body

Sarah Meehan O'Callaghan

Routledge
Taylor & Francis Group
LONDON AND NEW YORK

Designed cover image: Getty

First published 2027
by Routledge
4 Park Square, Milton Park, Abingdon, Oxon OX14 4RN

and by Routledge
605 Third Avenue, New York, NY 10158

*Routledge is an imprint of the Taylor & Francis Group, an Informa business*



*British Library Cataloguing in Publication Data*
A catalogue record for this book is available from the British Library

ISBN: 978-1-032-83497-9 (hbk)
ISBN: 978-1-032-83496-2 (pbk)
ISBN: 978-1-003-50962-2 (ebk)

DOI: 10.4324/9781003509622

Typeset in Times New Roman
by Taylor & Francis Books

For A.

# Contents

# Figure

# Acknowledgements

As this book grew out of the work of my previous PhD, I would like to acknowledge my then supervisors. Thank you to Jean-Philippe Imbert, Francesca Counihan, and Medb Ruane for all their input and support. I would also like to thank Carol Owens and Olga Cox Cameron for their input into this process and inspiration in sustaining 'the pilgrim' staff of Lacanian scholarship. Thanks also to Ian Parker and the editorial team at Routledge for their engagement with my work. I would also like to recognise the ongoing work of the psychoanalytic organisations APPI and ICLO for their rigorous engagement with Lacanian studies and for providing me with many thought-provoking opportunities in these matters.

# Series Preface for Sarah Meehan O'Callaghan's *Psychoanalysing Mind-Body Narratives Through Beckett and Artaud: The Trauma of the Body*

There is a convenient fiction circulating in caricature representations of Lacanian psychoanalysis, that the dissolving of instinctual processes into language in Lacan's work leads to a neglect of the corporeal bedrock of human existence. All the talk about signifiers, we are sometimes told, means that the elemental sexual stuff of the unconscious is turned into an idealist postmodern mish-mash of linguistic tropes. Here is a book to put that misunderstanding of developments in psychoanalysis – wishful thinking that is more of the realm of the imaginary than anything else – to bed, to show it rests not only on a misreading of Lacan's own return to Freud, but also rests on a misrecognition of the meaning of Lacanian psychoanalytic engagement with the work of two of the most important literary figures who are sometimes themselves glossed as 'postmodern', Samuel Beckett and Antonin Artaud.

This book traces an epistemology of the body as it intersects with subjectivity, showing that the traumatic and alienating dimension of embodiment has always been a key concern of Lacanian psychoanalysis. What this interdisciplinary book does so effectively is to take seriously the symbolic coordinates through which the human being as speaking being becomes human, social, and to show how that supposed knowledge of the body is located, cannot but be located in the shocking, disruptive, real of our material existence.

The experience of the body as ontological trauma for the human subject is explored and deconstructed through a reading of the works of Beckett and Artaud, in such a way as to harness insights from critical cultural and disability studies, those touching on the real of illness and pain. We thus learn about the role of the symbolic and the limits of mind-body dualism. It is here that the too-often normative and normalizing theory and practice of psychoanalysis, its symbolic status, can be interrogated, challenged by the real of the anomalous body, of the body that suffers from acute alterity. We are brought face to face with theatres of cruelty and of the absurd, motifs that have always been present in the Freudian image of the irredeemably tragic nature of human subjectivity, one that is always present in the clinic, but which has been most effectively expressed and theorized in literature.

Psychoanalytic clinical and theoretical work circulates through multiple intersecting antagonistic symbolic universes. This series opens connections between different cultural sites in which Lacanian work has developed in distinctive ways, in forms of work that question the idea that there could be single correct reading and application. The Lines of the Symbolic in Psychoanalysis series provides a reflexive reworking of psychoanalysis that transmits Lacanian writing from around the world, steering a course between the temptations of a metalanguage and imaginary reduction, between the claim to provide a god's eye view of psychoanalysis and the idea that psychoanalysis must everywhere be the same. And the elaboration of psychoanalysis in the symbolic here grounds its theory and practice in the history and politics of the work in a variety of interventions that touch the real

Ian Parker
Manchester Psychoanalytic Matrix

# Introduction

## On Not Knowing the Body

This book explores a question of knowledge concerning the human body through the works of two prominent 20th-century writers, Antonin Artaud (1896–1948) and Samuel Beckett (1906–1989), with a particular, but not exclusive, focus on their dramatic work. It asserts that a study of the body in their work, as that which reveals the body as an ontological trauma, can shed light on problematic narratives concerning the relation of body and mind that circulate in the socio-cultural imaginary. We shall see that acquiring knowledge of the body may be somewhat of an impossible quest, not entirely unlike the corporeal project of Antonin Artaud, a so-called failed theatre practitioner. Yet, I hope that, at the very least, this impossibility will be exposed as such, not as an ideal of transcendence, and that this approach will lead to the possibility of seeing the body differently. Ultimately, at the centre of this book is the fundamental and inalienable fact that being a human being involves inhabiting a body, a material frame through which we live our lives. We do not simply have a body but are also composed of it as an intrinsic and immanent element of our existence. However, when it comes to our relation to the body, we are not masters in our own homes. This perspective is the legacy of Freud, who situated the unconscious as central to our experience as human beings and decentred self-knowledge as the domain of rationality. Lacan's paradigm of the divided subject remains faithful to this idea, proposing that at any given time we are not in a position of absolute knowledge of ourselves as subjects. Fundamentally, there is something of ourselves that is structurally unknowable. I extend this idea to include the body, in that something of the body is unconscious, or perhaps aspects of our relationship to it. As subjects with bodies, we both are and have a body at the same time. I argue that this paradox of being and having a body is conflictual, traumatic and non-harmonious; indeed, we are never at one with our bodies, though we strive to be.

The question of knowledge lies at the heart of this exploration and considers what it is possible to learn about the problematics of the body through the medium, in particular but not exclusively, of the authors' theatrical works. I say problematics, given that the body that we speak of is not

DOI: 10.4324/9781003509622-1

something that we can take for granted as if it refers to something stable, unchanging and substantive. This ambiguity is what makes a study of the body both challenging and productive, as it is within the very elaboration of a question that the body, in all its complexity, takes shape. Both authors engage with the nature of embodiment, albeit at times indirectly, and grapple in their artistic work with the limits of representation in which the body is situated. Although I will refer to the representation of the body, by representation I also imply that which cannot be seen of the body but exists as a bodily trace within the text or performance. A central and complex point in this book is that a bodily trace can be understood by identifying an orientation for each author vis-à-vis the object a, the object cause of desire, as existing within the mise-en-scène of the theatrical or literary work. The object a is that intangible remainder of the collision of language with the body and is manifest through the bodily phenomena of an other, such as the gaze and the voice. Its relation to the body is important here. These attributes of the body that can trigger desire do not have a specular image, even though they distort the field of the visible (McGowan, 2007). We will be considering this idea both from the point of view of the authors, identifying a fundamental position regarding what I call the trauma of the body, a structural component of embodiment, and also how the object a within theatre may function for the spectator. In this sense, the nature of spectatorship is also significant as a place from which the body is seen, or not seen. Therefore, the context of subjectivity is paramount in considering these epistemological questions within this book, as it is a prism through which many things become distorted, including knowledge.

The human being has a blind spot concerning the body of another, and this 'other' is also one's self. To put this another way, the visual spectacle of the body cannot tell us as much as we sometimes think about the nature of who or what we are looking at. In considering this idea, we can ask: what are the limits of knowability regarding the body of another or indeed ourselves? What, indeed, is the purpose and consequence of asking this question? These questions shall be elaborated in detail in Chapters 1, 2, and 3 of the first part of the book, The Epistemology of the Body, and then analysed in Part Two in Chapters 4–7, The Body of Drama. Part 3, The Body Between Being and Non-Being, then takes up the body's relation to being. For the moment, it is enough to consider that something does not add up, is misaligned, or out of focus, regarding not only the visual field of the body but also what can be said or understood of it in the context of multi-modal meaning structures, disciplines, and practices. This asymmetry of relating (or knowing) comes to the fore in many particular and ubiquitous circumstances where communication is necessary to relay mental and physical states to another, or indeed, ourselves. These fields include psychotherapy, medical settings, and academic and scientific disciplines that interrogate the nature of embodiment and day-to-day social engagements. What happens, for example, when someone has a disease that is not yet understood or is "undocumented", as Anna Mollow (2018) puts it, and therefore lacks signifiers with which to describe the symptoms in the body within the context of a medical consultation room or outside? For although the signifiers we may use in this scenario may be our own descriptions, or our own words or metaphors for what is taking place in the body, without symbolic recognition, they do not hold the same meaning or quite hit the mark as more accepted symbols of bodily distress.

In this book, when speaking about mind-body narratives, I refer to cultural conceptions of the body-mind relation that are built on simplifications or erroneous assumptions of what constitutes body and mind and that filter down to the everyday lived experience of people with bodies or minds that have come into focus. In counteracting these narratives, I emphasise bodily states or physical manifestations that deviate from and challenge cultural narratives of the ideal body, such as disability, impairment, and a general not working out or an inherent failure of the body. This accent on anomaly is drawn from both my own experience of living with a disability and from the works of Beckett and Artaud, which have spoken to me about the body and its existential conundrums. It is challenging to take the subject out of the object of enquiry, but this is also a critical part of research—that is, to recognise one's own prejudices and biases and attempt to surpass finding the answers we want to find. Nonetheless, the accent in this book, chosen on alterity, is not an accident, even if it is born of accident or contingency. This is by way of saying there is something really interesting and important at work concerning the representation of alterity, or specifically bodily alterity, in the works of Beckett and Artaud, and this appreciation may be heightened if the spectator has experienced something of this corporeal alienation. I propose that all individuals/subjects in a Lacanian sense experience this alienation, but some experience it more than others, or sooner than others, particularly in the case of those living with chronic illness and disability. The cultural imaginary generates images of the ideal body that are often associated with qualities such as productivity, functionality, oneness, reproduction, and mastery. By contrast, states of impairment, bodily suffering, and pain are often denied or repudiated, or explanations are cast that place the onus on the psychology of the person experiencing these states. In this book, I expose the notion of the ideal body as a fantasy structure of the unconscious in which lack, impossibility, and trauma are veiled by an illusion of mastery. Furthermore, I propose that this fantasy is structural to the desire 'not to know' something about the body, or to a passion for ignorance concerning its complexity.

In attempting to think differently about the body as a consequence of the dialogue between psychoanalysis and the works of Beckett and Artaud, it is not my aim here to propose a paradigm that may inadvertently form yet another ideal (or narrative) in the place of the gap in knowledge constitutive of the body. In other words, I do not wish to propose a theoretical proposition of alternate embodied states as some sort of crip-utopia, which undermines the difficult reality of those living with difference, such as a construction of a non-normative paradigm where difference is reduced to sameness. In other words, all theory runs the risk of becoming yet another narrative, another plug in the gap of knowledge concerning the Real and the nature of being where difference or singularity is neutralised by a certain generality. This reduction to sameness is often done in an attempt to engender equality, whether this is in the disability area or the non-normative sexuality one. Similarly, Mitchell and Snyder argue in *The Biopolitics of Disability* (2015) that well-meaning attempts to deconstruct the stigma and marginalisation of differential embodiments by aligning everyone as inherently disabled or temporarily able-bodied (an argument within disability studies) actually dissipates the radical potential of these physical states and the particularities of living with impairment. We should be suspicious of utopic theoretical claims, including those that have the best interests of the marginalised at heart, as can occur in the discourse of human rights, where critical difference is often elided in favour of equality. What sometimes gets lost in these socio-political debates is that to be of equal value does not imply homogeneity.

Despite this caveat, the tensions that arise from this engagement situate a dialogue within the maelstrom of ideas that is the historically enduring body–mind (or, more traditionally, mind–body) problematic. In this book, these signifiers are expanded through a conception of the unconscious as the phenomenon that subverts the desire to know and the traditional binary between these terms. This also raises the issue of the body's relationship to the unconscious, which is not an easy question to answer but essential to consider in light of how the body and alterations to the organism affect the psyche.

## The Body Matters

In this book, I take the view that the body is not a static entity but a phenomenon that, upon investigation, yields to an understanding of fluidity, instability, and immanent heterogeneity. This is in keeping with the post-conventional approach, in which "all categories are slippery, fluid, heterogeneous, deeply intersectional, and thus resistant to definition" (Shildrick, 2009, p. 4). In this light, I contend that to have a body, as a human being, is to experience heterogeneity from within, as the experience of being different from ourselves, immanently alienated, embodied as an Other. We exist as the body and in relation to it (or indeed, as that very relation). Thus, the body is not something self-evident, strictly material, nor merely a reflection of the mind as a symmetrical counterpart. This critique allows for a more complex account of what it means to exist with the body and the potential to challenge simplistic narratives that deny the inherently traumatic dimensions of embodiment. These more simplistic accounts of body and mind are often found in the guise of popular discourses such as the cult of positive thinking (addressed by Barbara Ehrenreich in *Smile and Die* (2010)), therapies such as cognitive behavioural therapy, and psychoanalytic discourse where hysteria can become the catchall for somatic complaints – what Julia Segal refers to as the predominance of a belief in mind over matter, where a healthy mind presupposes a healthy body (J. Segal, personal communication, 6 October 2014). I argue that this predominance of understanding embodiment through the influence of the 'mind' is a response to the tension generated by a gap in knowledge concerning the body. This gap is structural to the subjectivity of the human being and not merely a consequence of a lack of empirical investigation. I develop this idea through Lacan's account of the Real as the gap in knowledge that can never be completely bridged through meaning systems. Although it is true that empiricism is hugely important in certain physical matters, particularly in the medical and scientific domains, from a psychoanalytic perspective, it does not have the same place as it does in science. This is due to the emphasis that psychoanalysis places on the function of language within the perimeters of subjectivity and the place given to what cannot be accounted for by objective and empirical means. The subject of the unconscious always elides the more tangible structures of empirical methods that adhere to principles of measurement and quantification. Psychoanalysis is interested in truth but this is a truth distinguished from knowledge in the scientific sense. As Derek Briton (2002) argues, science must exclude the truth of the Real in order to make knowledge possible (paragraph 6).

If truth is located in the Real, how do we express or capture it? The Lacanian Real is that which resists representation; it exists in a domain that is never fully outside language but resistant to it. Although some may argue that the Real is outside language, given that it is a function of language as a system or set of signifiers, in some respects, it cannot be completely separate from it. Distinctions between inside and outside are problematised in Lacan's work, as seen in his use of topology to elucidate the structure of the subject and the non-linear properties of the unconscious. Fundamentally, then, and in keeping with the theme of spatial paradox, this book addresses the gap in knowledge that I argue exists concerning the body by investigating it as a hole in knowledge, rather than replacing it with certainty or creating an empirical product. Although paradoxically, this book is a product, but not one that proffers closure.

In the dramatic work/writings under discussion, I contend that there is a possibility for the spectator to have an ethical encounter regarding the body. Although it is important to address the particularities of alienation experienced by certain subjects in relation to the body, it is not only through finding meaning that alienation is eased, but paradoxically, it can be through the encounter with a disruption of sense that a moment of alternate perception can be generated. We need the imaginary to be shaken up before we can glimpse beneath the defences that support it. Instead of attempting to fix the discord inherent to subjectivity and the body,, the presentation of this discord confronts the viewer with something difficult to face, perhaps even something unconscious, repressed from the habitual imaginary structures of reality.

## Art and Psychoanalysis

An assumption in this book is that, while the domains of literature and psychoanalysis encounter tensions in application, obviously, when dealing with literature, we are not relating to an active speaking subject as in the psychoanalytic clinic. Nonetheless, they are not entirely separate fields.

As a consequence of this assumption, the structure of this book is dialectical, creating a dialogue among psychoanalytic studies, theatre studies, disability studies, and the work of Artaud and Beckett. Ultimately, although the epistemology of the body varies across these disciplines and fields, the question of knowledge remains constant. As this book is informed by Lacanian psychoanalysis, the function or status of knowledge has particular import. In *Knowing Nothing: Staying Stupid*, Nobus and Quinn (2005) refer to the difference between knowledge acquisition in ordinary discourse and a psychoanalytic appraisal of this moment as an "epistemological fall" (p. 3)—acquiring knowledge can make us more stupid, as I understand it, if we think we have plugged the trauma of the unknown. That is, from a psychoanalytic point of view, there is a tension in any study that concerns itself with the production of knowledge about a particular lack of knowledge, in this case, the body.

Furthermore, how can we know something about what we do not know when what we do not know is a structural and pivotal point of our existence? This paradox of knowledge is especially pertinent to the present study, where subjectivity is at the fore. In this sense of the ambiguity of knowledge production, there is also a tension in forming interpretations regarding dramatic or artistic works, as the web of meaning, the play of signifiers used to convey information, is always involved in transmission. In this book, I attempt to underline and indeed draw out this tension in order to demonstrate the productivity of encountering the lack in the Other or in other words, the points at which meaning fails. For I argue, it is at these points that something of the body as an ontological phenomenon also emerges. In this approach, I aim to avoid reductive applications of theory to its object of study and to foster a more lively engagement with psychoanalytic concepts and the phenomenological qualities of the theatrical works under review. In other words, the plays under investigation cannot simply be explored as representations of theory but as active agents of its critique. In thinking of the dynamics of application, I would like to draw on an idea espoused by Laura Cull (2012) in "Performance as Philosophy". Cull points out that "Etymologically, 'apply' comes from the Latin *applicare*, which simply means 'to bring things in contact with one another'" (p. 21). From this point of view, analysing a theatrical work is not a hermeneutics in which we extract essentialist meanings inscribed within the play; rather, both theory and its subject are altered by the encounter. As Cull argues, performance is a form of thinking; it is philosophy in action and therefore does not exist in isolation from theory. In some respects, to separate theory from performance is to enact a Cartesian approach to the study of theatre: there is the mind (theory) and the body (performance). When in practice the body (mind) also thinks through movement, the action on stage is not simply representing reality as theory, but recreating it, adding another dimension.

Indeed, it must be said that the 'application' of psychoanalysis to the artistic and literary domain is not without its tensions. Apart from grappling with Lacan's concepts, which change over time and destabilise the reader in terms of meaning, we also face the issue of knowledge and the question of reading for the unconscious in a non-clinical setting. That is to say, the potentially obvious point is that the artistic space is not a setting in which one person speaks to another for the purpose of analysis, nor is it one in which we may encounter parapraxis, slips of the tongue, or bungled actions. In other words, the phenomenon of transference, that vector of love and projection between two speaking beings, is not in play. This raises the question of whether reading for the unconscious in artworks is even possible. I would propose an analogue system in which we do not deal with the unconscious directly but can infer unconscious formations through motifs, repetitions, and the function of language. However, artworks themselves can be products of the unconscious, ways of inventing solutions to enigmatic questions, but we cannot decipher them as if there were a definitive meaning behind the scenes.

While the distinction between the clinical and the artistic space may be non-reducible, it is clear from the work of Lacan and Freud that theatre, art and literature infuse the space of psychoanalysis. What we classify as psychoanalytic theory is already somewhat a product of a certain degree of literary/dramatic analysis. We do not have to go far to see the influence of theatre and drama within the theoretical trajectory of psychoanalysis, such as *Oedipus Rex* in the Oedipus complex, *Hamlet*, desire, grief and the fundamental fantasy in *Seminar VI, Desire and its Interpretation* (1958–1959), the Claudel trilogy of *Seminar VIII, Transference* (1960–1961) and Antigone as an ethical paradigm of not giving ground to desire and the function of beauty in dramatic art in *Seminar VII, The Ethics of Psychoanalysis* (1959–1960). Literature and the arts provide the means for Lacan and Freud, each in their own way, to stage specifically the "tragic dimension of psychoanalysis" (Lacan, 1997, p. 291). Interestingly, in *The New Black*, psychoanalyst Darian Leader describes turning to literature to explore the nature of subjective experiences regarding depression, loss, and melancholia and the corresponding dearth of information on this experience in the scientific field. As he says: "It then occurred to me that perhaps the scientific literature on mourning that I had been searching for was simply all literature" (Leader, 2008, p. 6). It is certainly true that qualities and 'truths' of subjective experience are often better documented through the arts rather than through so-called empirical sciences and, indeed, the discourse of psychoanalytic theory. Literary poetics of expression and the expanses of metaphor may succeed in transmitting subjective experience that other modes of expression may stifle (Meehan O'Callaghan, 2024). What is critically important to bear in mind is that while paradoxically, the clinic and artistic space are undoubtedly different realms of encounter, literature and fiction are as integral to the practice and theory of psychoanalysis as is the clinical case study, which indicates how discursive binaries of theory and practice are suspect, at least. This suggests that these explorations within the artistic domain regarding the body may ultimately have clinical consequences, despite the clear demarcation of the spaces.

## Comparative Context

The comparative analysis of the dramatic works of Artaud and Beckett entails a large corpus. Both authors were novelists, playwrights, and poets, and in Artaud's case, an actor. Artaud had several screen appearances as an actor, as well as playing the central role of Count Cenci in his play *The Cenci*. Consequently, the range of writings and literary works is substantial, indeed, with the exception of Artaud's produced dramatic work. Beckett, in particular, has been the most prolific when it comes to the stage, with a body of drama that completely dwarfs that of Artaud. Increasingly, Beckett's short stories and prose texts have been adapted for the stage with recent productions such as *Watt* by Barry McGovern (2019), *Company* by Sarah Jane Scaife (2018) and *No's Knife* by Lisa Dwan (2017). These recent adaptations situate Beckett's dense novelistic worlds within a visual space where the transition from reader to spectator takes place. As the focus of this book is predominantly, although not exclusively, drama, not all of each author's writings feature in this analysis.

By focusing more specifically on the context of dramatic texts and performance, a more coherent and thorough approach to the subject becomes possible. Nonetheless, transitions are made from particular writings and prose texts when relevant to themes, styles, and motivations deemed to be pertinent to the topic of the body within the dramatic context. The exploration of transitions from text to stage emphasises movements inherent to representing the body with the subsequent implications for representation, embodiment, and spectatorship. For example, Beckett wrote *Waiting for Godot* after completing the trilogy with *The Unnamable*, where, in certain respects, the process of narration was exhausted in the very act of that narration and where the interior space of the novel is plumbed to its very limits. The theatre of Artaud's theoretical project, although ornate and perspicacious in its formulation, is deemed to have been a failure when put into practice on the stage.

The invention of a body-orientated theatre is very clearly evident in Artaud's manifesto for a Theatre of Cruelty. To fully appreciate his vision and given the scarcity of staged productions of his work, it is necessary to investigate his theoretical writings on theatre. Artaud is also a popular figure of avant-garde iconography, an emblem of poetic martyrdom, a romanticised madman whose writings on the sufferings of his own body and his relationship to language have interested many a philosopher and literary critic, including Foucault, Derrida, Deleuze, and Kristeva. Additionally, Artaud's art and the drawings he created at the psychiatric institution of Rodez between 1938 and 1945 are of great interest to studies on the nature of psychosis, such as *Incandescent Alphabets: Psychosis and the Enigma of Language* (2016/2018) by Annie Rogers.

The comparative analysis of Artaud and Beckett provides a multifaceted lens within which different angles on the body come to the fore. The difference in the styles of each dramatist can be assessed in the context of understanding the relationship to meaning in each dramatic work and its implications for the field of spectatorship. Although studies of the alterity of the body have been conducted on the works and writings of these authors, a comparative analysis of the body that posits the unconscious as central to the investigation has important cross-disciplinary implications. We shall see in the following chapters how the comparison of dramatic works elucidates and illuminates a thematics of the body in a way that a study of a single author would not. I propose that there are distinctive differences in how Beckett and Artaud represent and relate to the body and these differences can shed light on the complexity of being and having a body.

In order to appreciate the nuances of this comparison, I will show over the next few chapters that, psychoanalytically speaking, the body is a paradox of the speaking being; that is, we are subjects who speak and create meaning symbolically (the Symbolic and the Imaginary) and who also feel at the level of the flesh (the Real), in ways that are often beyond language, or at least beyond expression in its entirety. This paradox between being and having creates conflict at the level of egoic identifications and generates anxiety, as the Real component of the body (in Lacanian terms, the organism) lies outside cognitive knowledge and demands management in day-to-day contexts and during times of extreme stress and tension. From an imaginary perspective, we can be caught in a hall of mirrors where potential identifications seduce us into the illusion of corporeal wholeness or unity. This book demonstrates that the conflict inherent to embodiment and its paradoxical status is dramatised within the work of Beckett and Artaud, albeit differently, and lived as a drama that plays out in the life of the human being.

Ultimately, through a study of their theatre as a predominant focus, we can learn something about the nature of this paradox and how attempts to express it fail in a way that ironically brings us closer to the truth of the relation between language, the body, and representation. Failure will thus be at the heart of this enquiry: the failure of the body as a trauma of existence, the intrinsic entropy of our flesh which haunts the neoliberal cultural imaginary of the whole and autonomous self, the failure of language to fully capture this reality, and failure as a theme in both authors' works. The juxtaposition of these two dramatists and authors allows us to see the nuances between their positions concerning a stance/orientation toward the body. So it is not only how the representation of the body challenges ideals of embodiment within their dramatic work that is at stake; contemplate, for example, the continuous appearance of incapacitated bodies in Beckett's work and the emphasis on the drive to physical catharsis as a means of transcending language in Artaud's vision of the Theatre of Cruelty. Also present is the epistemological question they appear to be grappling with through the trope of the suffering body.

A question that may arise is why I have predominantly chosen dramatic works rather than their complete works to illustrate or interrogate questions concerning mind-body narratives and the body. Apart from the logistics of pursuing this endeavour and the sheer magnitude of writings by both authors, there is something about theatre that is of particular interest when interrogating the representation of the body, which often leads to the assumption that the body is very present, real, and embodied as performance. While this is not completely untrue, the presumption of presence should be questioned, the pursuit of which can lead us to some very interesting insights concerning the limits of representation as a function of spectatorship and the role of the imaginary in the structural composition of the body. That is, the body may be present on stage, but present to whom? There is a certain reception that needs to be questioned. Furthermore, the very employment of the stage by both Beckett and Artaud as a means to express dimensions of their work suggests something at the level of meaning and otherness that further elaborates on their stance or orientation toward the body. In other words, theatre addresses or provokes the spectator in a particular way that is different to the interiority generated by reading a novel. It can be said that the other (the spectator) serves a particular function through the theatrical modality as a receptacle for the witnessing and interpretation of a narrative. In theatre, there is a literal audience rather than an imagined one (as with a novel), although the audience is always in part imagined even if it is present. Certainly, the role of the stage as sending messages to, or addressing, the other, and the category of audience reception, are of great importance in understanding Artaud's orientation vis-à-vis meaning, language, the body, and Otherness. The Theatre of Cruelty was an invention conceived to have a physical effect on the audience, waking them from the slumber of Western rationalism and psychological realism, and provoking a catharsis that was not Aristotelian but Dionysian: the effect was not about order but disorder, a revolt of the unconscious.

In my investigation, I consider how Artaud's quest for a space beyond language in his corporeal theatre was infiltrated by a desire to be free of the conflict inherent to mind–body dualism, a conflict perpetuated by language's conventions. Artaud's quest was motivated by what I call the trauma of the body, a concept influenced by a Lacanian account of trauma as ontological and that demands further elaboration in the coming chapters. Therefore, with this study of theatre and the later emphasis on spectatorship, I begin with a question of the Real of the body (the living felt body outside of knowledge) and develop it through the travails of the imaginary and symbolic (body as perceived, imagined in theatre), as fundamental to a perspective on paradoxes inherent to the aesthetic encounter. In other words, how do we read for the trauma of the body in theatre when aspects of it are beyond language and meaning?

While in this book we are focusing on the theme of the body in an almost phenomenological way, that is, as an entity present and absent within the drama, I do not concentrate in-depth on historical factors pertaining to the context and background of the authors. Nonetheless, certain elements are important in situating these authors together and painting a picture of the symbolic and social factors surrounding their work and epoch. An interesting connection between these two authors (who, as Matthew Melia (2007) points out, never actually met) is the director and actor Roger Blin. Blin directed Artaud's *The Cenci* (1925), Beckett's *Endgame* (1957), and *Waiting for Godot* (1953), thereby establishing a link between the work of these authors, at least in the productive context.

In his famous category of the "Theatre of the Absurd," Martin Esslin (1961) included Artaud and Beckett as practitioners of this style of "New Theatre," in which the events on stage (as forms) transcend the words spoken:[1] "The Theatre of the Absurd has renounced arguing about the absurdity of the human condition; it merely presents it in being—that is, in terms of concrete stage images. This is the difference between the approach of the philosopher and that of the poet" (1961, paragraph, 21). Esslin's categorisation offers an interesting historical framework for juxtaposing the stylistic similarities and differences among the various dramatic works, and it situates the dramatists in a context concerned with meaning. According to Esslin, absurdity is a "sense of the senselessness of life, of the inevitable devaluation of ideals, purity, and purpose" (ibid, intro, paragraph 18). In this context, the stage abandons the linear movement of textual narrative in favour of a style of performance that shows in aesthetic form 'how it is'. Although Esslin connects absurdity as related to particular societal conditions and a type of 'metaphysical anguish' within existence, from the perspective of this book, we can view this concept differently. In other words, feelings of anguish or absurdity are rooted in the state of embodied existence as a structural precondition of existence. It is not simply the meaning of life that is at stake for us as a metaphysical question, but the very senselessness of physiological processes and bodily contingencies, which radically colour our perspective on life. Our very identities are infused by the backdrop of the body, and hence, the relation between the body and meaning is deeply complex. I will return to this idea over the coming chapters.

## The Structure of the Book

Given that the 'subject' (as in subject matter) of the body is not simply a statement but also a question (what is a body?), this is a question that I address in this book as open-ended and not conclusive. At the level of language and, by extension, subjective experience, the human body is not a static, unchanging phenomenon but is influenced by culture, prevailing trends in discourse, and the aesthetics of becoming—the drive to always improve, modify, alter the body in some way. As a result, representations and, indeed, experiences of it change over time. That said, there is also something constant about the body, which is the conflict at the heart of our relationship with it and the paradox of being that engaging it as a question presents.

Given the dialectical approach of this book, in which a psychoanalytic account of the body informs the analysis of the body in the dramatic works and vice versa, it is divided into three parts: Part 1: The Epistemology of the Body; Part 2: The Drama of the Body; Part 3: The Body between Being and Non-Being. The key point is that this is an analysis of mind–body narratives *through* the theatre of Beckett and Artaud and not *in* as would be the case with a direct interpretative approach to this subject.

Furthermore, as theatre is an art form comprised of both text and performance, I have adopted an approach that includes theory concerning the reception of performance as well as that which concerns the texts. It is not possible to speak of theatre without taking this dual aspect into account, even if this results in inevitable tensions or deficits of application. By this, I mean that wherever possible, I attended performances of the dramatic works in question, but some were not available as a live performance, though accessible in pre-recorded form. This is particularly relevant to the plays of Artaud, which I have never attended a performance or enactment of, but this is not surprising due to the lack of staged productions.

Given the parameters of this book's trajectory within the work of Beckett and Artaud, the elaboration of Lacan's ideas regarding the body is far from exhaustive. As regards terminology, concepts such as the object a are defined according to a particular timeframe or seminar. Thus, it is important to note that these definitions are provisional on the timeframe in question and that these concepts may change or develop in later seminars. However, the main focus is the relevance of the concepts to a reading of the body, rather than the change in Lacan's thinking per se, although this is also noted where possible.

Additionally, the term object a was not intended to be translated, as is the case with jouissance. As such, it is not possible to have completely satisfactory or conclusive definitions of these terms, but the position they occupy in the methodology is supported by Lacan's words and secondary criticism. As the method and application are dialectical, in that the dramatic texts may also inform Lacanian theory regarding the body, these ideas remain open to further interprctation or elaboration in this book. As I have indicated already, in order to 'read' for the trauma of the body in a theatrical context, the body itself must come under inspection as a question, a signifier rather than a destination. Let us begin with the question of the body.

## Note

1 Esslin places Artaud's theoretical writings within the category of the absurd and not specifically the relatively few plays under his name.

## References

Artaud, A. (1935/1999). *The Cenci.* Collected works of Antonin Artaud Volume 4. (V. Corti, Transl.).pp. 212–221). London: John Calder.

Artaud, A. (1938/1958). *The theatre and its double* (M.C. Richards, Transl.). New York: Grove Press.

Lacan, J. (1975–1976). *The seminar of Jacques Lacan, book XXIII. Joyce and the sinthome.* (C. Gallagher, Transl.) Unpublished.

Beckett, S. (1953/2006). Waiting for Godot. In *Samuel Beckett. The complete dramatic works* (pp. 7–89). Croydon: Faber & Faber.

Beckett, S. (1953/1978). *The unnamable.* New York: Grove Press.

Beckett, S. (1958). Molloy. In *S. Beckett: Three novels, Molloy, Malone Dies, The Unnamable* (pp. 1–170). New York: Grove Press.

Briton, D. (2002). The truth is that which runs after the truth. *University of Stirling.* 2–4 July. Retrieved 29 November 2019 from http://www.leeds.ac.uldeducol/documents/00002060.htm.

Cull, L. (2012). Performance as philosophy: Responding to the problem of 'application'. *Theatre Research International*, 37 (1), 20–27.

Ehrenreich, B. (2010). *Smile or die: How positive thinking fooled America and the world.* London: Granta Books.

Lacan, J. (1958–1959). *Desire and its interpretation: Seminar VI.* (C. Gallagher, Transl.) Dublin: Unpublished.

Lacan, J. (1959–1960/1997). *Seminar VII. The ethics of psychoanalysis.* (J. Alain-Miller, Ed., & D. Porter, Transl.) London: Norton & Company.

McGowan, T. (2007). *The real gaze. Film theory after Lacan.* Albany: New York Press.

Meehan O'Callaghan, S. (2024). A question of beauty: Lacan's seventh seminar and the oblique ethics of an aesthetic encounter. *Lacunae*, 26, Winter-Spring. Appi.

Melia, M. (2007). *Architecture and cruelty: The writings of Artaud, Beckett and Genet.* Unpublished thesis. London.

Mitchell, D.T & Snyder, S. L (2015). *The biopolitics of disability: Neoliberalism, ablenationalism, and peripheral embodiment*. USA: University of Michigan Press.

Nobus, D. & Quinn, M. (2005). *Knowing nothing, staying stupid: Elements of a psychoanalytic epistemology.* Sussex: Routledge.

Rogers, A. (2016/2018). *Incandescent alphabets: Psychosis and the enigma of language.* New York: Routledge.

Shildrick, M. (2009). *Dangerous discourses of disability, subjectivity and sexuality.* London: Palgrave Macmillan.

# Part I

# The Epistemology of the Body

Part I of this book assumes the body as an epistemological phenomenon rather than something we know a priori. Before investigating the trauma of the body in the works of Beckett and Genet, the first three chapters build a case for understanding why the body is an ontological trauma and how this perspective can challenge problematic mind–body narratives that deny the fundamental unknowability of the body in its entirety.

Chapter 1 outlines why the body itself is an open-ended question, both in theoretical terms and as a motif in the work of the authors. Chapter 2 expands on the topic of ableism as an overarching category of how narratives of the body/mind often work to stigmatise and alienate those with differential embodiment. Chapter 3 then provides an antithesis to these narratives by constructing a theory of the body in which mind over matter is problematised as a binary that forecloses the complexity of the very terms 'body' and 'mind'.

DOI: 10.4324/9781003509622-2

Chapter 1

# The Question of the Body

It is said that there are only two certainties in life: death and taxes. However, another thing is certain about the existence of human beings, at least so far in the history of humanity: there is no being or subject, no existence, without a body. It is arguably the unstable ground of being. In order to live as human beings, we must possess some sort of corporeal frame that holds the breath of our existence. From what could be conceived of as a materialist secular perspective, this is where our conflicts begin because to exist as a human being is to inhabit a body subject to inner drives, determinants, and contingencies that cause traumatic disturbances in lived experience. Human beings are embodied subjects who exist as a function of the world and are therefore also subject to the contingencies of this world as bodily events. In some respects, the body might be all there is, and all that we are reduced to at the beginning and the end of our lives. However, from the perspective of the psychoanalytic divided subject, a paradox lies at the heart of embodiment. As subjects with an unconscious, we exist *through* the frame of corporeal materiality *and* as a relationship to the body (which psychoanalysis would suggest is not reducible to merely material flesh). In what I argue is a conflictual dichotomy, we both *are* and *have* a body and exist as subjects in the interstices of this contradiction. This implies, in fact, that our subjectivity is not reducible to our material reality, but is also a function of language and the symbolic structures within which we live.

In contemporary times, theories of mind–body relations have shifted away from the Cartesian split between mind and body. While Descartes's *cogito ergo sum* is the mantra that forms the bedrock of theorising against a split between psyche and soma, I contend in this book that we need to consider a divided ontology regarding our relation to the body. This idea is developed through tracing a theory of the body and being through Lacan and critiquing it through Beckett and Artaud, authors who clearly grapple with the body's boundaries, its relation to the self, and the depth and nature of being. Primarily, I argue that if we take the unconscious as central to the investigation of the body in the work of these authors, we can trace two differing ontological positionalities arising from a relation to the body as a central theme. In later chapters, I flesh this idea out in greater detail through an analysis of the

DOI: 10.4324/9781003509622-3

authors' works. For the moment, I will leave it here as a core background question that I will return to. I wish, however, to emphasise early on the ontological accent of this enquiry and how an originally epistemological investigation of the body becomes one that centres on the very primacy of being. I contend that the ontology of the body is marked by trauma—trauma in a Lacanian sense—with a view to disturbing conceptions of the body–mind relation as they can be unearthed in cultural narratives of embodiment, including those within psychoanalysis. These narratives often work to stigmatise or cover over the conflictual and traumatic dimension of the body, as narratives or stories can be ways of creating meaning and taming the enigma of the mind–body relation. In this sense, even narratives of trauma, which we can see proliferating in our times, may shield us from a disturbing excess at the heart of being. In order to conduct this ontological enquiry, it is necessary to consider the body as a question, an entity or term whose meaning we cannot take for granted but must be interrogated as an epistemological study. In the next chapter, I examine the nature of mind–body narratives within culture in more detail and explore why they are problematic; for now, I focus on what constitutes a body in the first place and why this is relevant to the work of Beckett and Artaud. Furthermore, in the drama of these writers, we will see that it is not simply a matter of how the body is represented on the stage, but rather a question for both authors, one that refracts theatrically and places demands of interrogation on the spectator. In other words, I think that both authors grapple with the essence of inhabiting a body in different ways and their theatre provides a means of containing and manifesting this struggle—a struggle that engages with the very essentials of being. Admittedly, this is a complex point and difficult to demonstrate, so it is necessary to navigate some lengthy theoretical issues concerning the body to set the stage for the analysis of the theatrical work in later chapters. I will ask a simple question to add more flesh to this idea at this juncture. Why would the body be a question for someone rather than something that is taken for granted or not even considered as the backdrop to the self? I suggest the question may arise when it becomes painfully present as an object of consciousness due to suffering, pain, or limitation of different kinds, including scenarios that cause affects and feelings that may not be specifically located in the body, but also manifest as suffering within the mind. The body is a source of limit points for the subject, limits that the human being invariably tries to transcend. When these limits come into focus, whether through extremes of endogenous pain or external restrictions such as imprisonment or environmental curtailment (think of Beckett's sparse landscapes and minimalist settings where the body is often trapped), the body itself often becomes a site of existential enquiry. Artaud's writings certainly give voice to this dual-aspect suffering and the porous boundaries between matter and mind—in fact, it can be argued that he attempts to transcend mind through matter by inventing a corporeal language in his writing and the Theatre of

Cruelty. For both Beckett and Artaud, apart from their own particular bodily sufferings, which could have rendered the body present as an existential conundrum, something that caused them to grapple with their very existence, it is clear that the question of the body–mind relation is also a philosophical one that manifests as an orientation or aesthetic concerning the body. That is, we can trace Cartesian (body-and-mind split) and post-Cartesian (attempt to undo this split) narratives of the self through their theatre. However, at the heart of these narratives or anti-narratives concerns an ambiguity about what the body actually is for the authors in question but also as a lived phenomenon. We cannot speak of mind–body relations with any coherence without asking what body we are speaking of.

## Fake Heading 1 – please remove at typesetting stage

### *What is a Body?*

Before I delve into the specifics of the orientation of the body in the dramatic works and some of the paradoxes it provokes, it is necessary to interrogate why the question of the body is so pertinent, why it would have been of such import for Beckett and Artaud, and what is at stake in such an epistemological enquiry. It might be too easy to say that both authors suffered hugely from the body, although they almost certainly did; Artaud had physical illnesses from a young age and was in the grip of an opium addiction for most of his adult life and Beckett suffered from somatic and psychical distress and his relatively short psychoanalysis with Bion is well known. Both authors have been referred to as having disabilities of sorts. However particular their individual experience was, I think it is more nuanced to consider how the more universal experience of suffering is localised in the trope of the suffering body in their work, a suffering that is not simply corporeal but existential, felt both psychically and physically, and is also something that extends beyond their individual lives through the signifiers of writing and drama. To put this more simply, while some people suffer more from the body than others, for all sorts of reasons we all suffer in and from the body. Some of our bodily experiences may be beyond our conscious appraisal. As a result of the opacity of our experiences, explanations for bodily phenomena often take the form of attributing a psychic reason to the cause of suffering —a somewhat top-down model of causation (the psychosomatic field) rather than investigating how the body itself impacts the mind (the somatopsychic angle of enquiry). To do this, however, we need to define the terms of the debate or understand why it is so complex to frame the body as a question in the first place. How do we even distinguish between the mind and body? We shall see that defining these terms is far from easy and brings us precariously close to what has been historically called the 'mind–body problem', a source of great speculative, biological, philosophical, and scientific enquiry for centuries.

And so we might ask: what is a body? We shall see that asking ourselves this question always raises the related question: what is a mind?[1] Using the logic of language, if there is an entity, the body, then it must be in relation to something that isn't the body, i.e. a mind or a psyche. Are there simply two entities, or registers of being, as in body and mind, or are we dealing with a much more complex phenomenon in which there are not simply two reciprocal poles of embodiment but something else outside this binary? What does asking the question about the nature of the body do for us, if anything? In some respects, these questions involve asking ourselves who we are and what we are, and, as the interrogations are predominantly psychoanalytic in nature, I would say that posing the question is more significant than providing a final answer. Desire is, after all, driven more by questions than by answers. A central argument in this book is that an exploration of the body does not lead to a definitive answer that can categorically signify the meaning of a body as some indisputable substance, nor can it deny it as a substance, but rather, we will encounter the means through which we come to know or interpret the body to be of central importance. In other words, how we know the body or how we relate to it in psychic fantasy and with the unconscious in mind is all part of embodied experience, even if it does not result in a signifier of wholeness to designate meaning. While defining the body might seem initially obvious—as in the body we are relating to is the one that we can see, touch, and feel, or the place from which we live in the world—from a Lacanian point of view, demarcating the boundaries of the body is not so clear-cut. There is a distinction to be made between the body as it relates to the signifier and the living or organic body. This distinction will be revisited in Chapter 3, where I examine a psychoanalytic account of the body more closely. According to Lacan in *Seminar XXIV, L'insu que Sait,* "We do not know what a living body is. It is an affair which for our part we have to leave to God" (Lesson 8: Wednesday 8 March 1977, p. 95). By living body, I think Lacan is referring here to the biological body, a term that is quite psychoanalytically complex when we take into account the impact of language on the materiality of the flesh, and whether, indeed, there is any primary physical substance. Colette Soler (1984) has pointed out that psychoanalysis has not brought much in the way of knowledge about the biological body. The body is a reality, but reality is a superstructure formed in part from the fictions of intra- and inter-psychic life. It is not a primary, given:

> To say that the body is a reality, means that the body is not primary. It means that one is not born with a body. In other words, I am saying that it is some reality, but in the sense that reality, since Freud, has a subordinate status: it is something which is constructed, which is secondary.
> (1984, paragraph 4)

Soler gives voice to a prevailing view in Lacanian psychoanalysis—the organism and the body are not the same thing. "There is a distinction to be made between the organism, the living being, on the one hand, and that which, on the other hand, is called the body" (Soler, p. 3). While I will leave this distinction here for the moment, my argument is that it is not so easy to separate the organism of the living being from the body we may refer to as the symbolic or imaginary body and that this distinction is not as clear as it might seem in Lacan's theory.

In our current times, the topic of the body as a construct rather than a biological given features strongly within many disciplines and fields, including theatre studies, gender studies, disability studies, philosophy, and psychotherapy, to name a few. However, before reading too much significance into this proliferation of research, as I said earlier, we need to ask: which body is being referred to when it comes into focus? In other words, is it a body assumed to be a physical substance that complements the mind in a causal exchange where one reflects the other, or is it a body that, independent of psychic phenomena, in Lacanian parlance, suffers, enjoys, or incurs events through the domain of the signifier? I would suggest that there is a certain tendency in psychotherapeutic modalities toward idealising the signification of the materiality of the body, or exalting it as a source of truth, in what Soler describes as the fashionable trend of localising the body therapeutically and analytically, evidenced by the proliferation of "physical therapies" or "body techniques" (1984, p. 1) where the body is a cipher of secrets and repressed traumas. In her view, these physical therapies, such as primal scream therapy and yoga, are techniques of the master signifier, ways of organising the subject into a particular symbolic order and taming the anxiety of the unknown and the Real of trauma. From this perspective, trauma, defined as the unassimilable effect of a past experience written on the body, can often be seen as a potential avenue for liberation and release. The rationale here is that if we can access the trauma that is inscribed upon the body, a liberation from the effect of this trauma can occur. Although it is true that the body often says more than we consciously realise and can reveal our real feelings and thoughts in many instances, for example, through body language, placing the concept of subjective truth in identity with the body is problematic. Perhaps we are dealing with two different registers, two different levels of truth. Another example of such corporeal idealisation is the idea of presence in theatre studies, interestingly, a possible influence of Artaud's emphasis on originality, where the body on stage signifies all that is present, alive, and current, happening now without mediation, as if we could access a greater truth of existence in this format of immediacy. The liveness of a dramatic performance, the happening now aspect before our eyes, can make the reception of the staged body appear as a pure phenomenological experience, in which the mediation of the spectator's gaze (the Real of subjectivity) is left out of the equation.

Nonetheless, despite the reductionist tendencies within certain theories of body studies, the increasing focus on corporeality and embodiment suggests a shift in the nature of considering what it means to be a human. James Berger (2004) describes this shift as the broad theoretical trend over the previous twenty years toward non-linguistic or more embodied forms of analysis, which he refers to as counter-linguistic turns, such as the 'somatic turn' in the field of disability studies and the 'outside of language' dimension of trauma studies. Another way of looking at this trend is that privileging the body as a subject of debate is a way of asking about the cause of being and of shifting the question of what drives our existence out of the metaphysical realm into a more material, physical, and possibly individualistic perspective on being. In chapter 3, I look more closely at the idea of cause and trauma as it concerns the body, through the Lacanian concept of the object a as the mythical object lost to the body in its very constitution through the collision with language. For the present, let us consider why the body's relation to the mind, and indeed the putative segmentation of a person into these two key components, has been a source of such enigma and controversy throughout time.

## *Mind–Body Problem*

The mind–body problem, as it is widely known, has existed for centuries and concerns the attempts to discern the nature of the relation between mind and body from scientific and philosophical perspectives. Is one causal of the other? Can they be reduced to the same substance? Where does consciousness originate in the brain? As Galadí (2023) points out, what is commonly referred to as the mind–body problem is often a conglomeration of multiple overlapping issues, including the 'hard problem' of consciousness (i.e. how does the brain give rise to subjective experience?). In fact, the philosophical 'problem', due to the backdrop of current neuroscientific research, has now been renamed as the 'mind–brain' problem. According to Mark Solms (2019), the way the question of causality is posed is a source of confusion, specifically whether the brain causes consciousness or whether neural correlates cause psychic phenomena. Solms argues that the brain does not cause consciousness any more than the liver creates bile. Solms is a proponent of 'dual-aspect monism' where both "body and mind are two appearances (aspects) of the same underlying thing" (2019)—critically, for neuropsychoanalysis, the mind cannot be reduced to the brain, though it is strongly related to it. In *The Feeling Brain* (2015), Solms argues for an integration of neuroscience and psychoanalysis in order to account for the subjective component of the brain within the scientific field. He argues that the brain is a feeling agent (it reflects on itself) and that this contingency has been overlooked by certain psychiatric and scientific, as well as neuropsychological, models of the mind.

While this book does not focus explicitly on the question of consciousness, nor does it attempt to solve the mind–body problem, which would be a lofty endeavour indeed, it incorporates conceptual avenues leading from it within the contours of identifying mind–body narratives, such as monism and duality, and how Beckett's and Artaud's drama reveal and critique them. In some respects, as we shall see, for Artaud, theatre was an attempt to solve the affectual discordance inherent to the subjective experience of having a body. While I think that all subjects experience this sense of discordance, some suffer from it more than others, and Artaud certainly falls into that category. There is an argument that duality is a pertinent aspect of subjective experience, in the sense that it seems there is a distinction between mind and body, because it *feels* that way, which doesn't mean they are separate or disconnected but that we have different qualitative experiences of a sense of fragmentation or disharmony between how we experience ourselves as thinking subjects and as subjects with a body. This would be in keeping with Solm's (2019) emphasis on affect as the "element form of consciousness". It also relates to Galadí's proposed dissolution of the problem of separation in the first place by, as he argues, uncovering the hidden identification of the mental with 'what I am' and the physical with 'what I am not' within Descartes' thought. Galadí shifts the terms of the debate from the opposition between the mental and the physical to a perceived duality based on being and not being:

> The key is to realize that I as a subject cannot avoid separating the universe into what I am and what I am not. 'What I am not' I know precariously, and this brings me to a scientific problem that is currently far from being solved.
>
> (2023, p. 16)

While Galadí's solution focuses on reassessing the terms of the debate in light of ontology and on undoing the problem by highlighting Descartes' hidden assumptions, it is interesting to note how attempts to define the difference or to make the connection between matter and mind have changed over time. While Descartes, in the seventeenth century, conjectured that animal spirits and the pineal gland were the means by which mind and body communicate, by the early twentieth century, Freud referred to ideational representatives as representing something of the body in the unconscious. Both Descartes and Freud, in different ways, were attempting to identify the pathway through which one part of the human being communicates to another, i.e. for Freud, with the concept of the drive, signals from bodily sensations become represented within the unconscious by a signifier, the ideational representative, which is not the sensation per se. Therefore, something in the psyche represents the body, or marks it as a trace in a way that we are not conscious of. It might be truer to say there is something represented in the unconscious that relates to the body, but it is not the body, at least as we know it in a discursive sense, as an actual, concrete entity. Freud's

(1923) conception of the ego as, first and foremost, a "bodily ego", posits the ego as a gateway between the internal sensations of the body and the intrapsychic representations of the external world. In this sense, the ego is a partial representative of the body without being reduced to it as a bodily substance, though it is, of course, born of this bodily substance and, I would argue, has a protective function in our emotional and physiological health.

For instance, diseases or illnesses that cause acute, chronic, or general pain or malaise will affect the ego and the narcissistic economy of the human subject. This is an important point to acknowledge and bears a relationship to Freud's point in *Mourning and Melancholia* (1917) that there may be a somatic component to 'toxic' feelings of melancholia. Melancholia can be induced by the direct effects of loss but also by a narcissistic and physical injury. Freud conjectured that the unconscious could speak through the body in the form of hysterical symptoms and introduced what we could call the idea of the speaking body, one of the key narratives, according to Anne Harrington (2008), of mind–body medicine in the twentieth century. While the psychoanalysts of the early twentieth century theorised the relationship between psychic symptoms, the body, and the realm of unconscious experience, the phenomenologists of the same century also took account of the different modes of perception pertaining to the more conscious experience of the body. In *The Phenomenology of Perception* (1945), Merleau-Ponty discusses the body's status as an object within the perceptual field. The disjunction of being and having is manifest in the paradoxical situation of the body, where the body is both subject and object of perception. In writing about the centrality of the body in subjective experience, he makes the critical point that we can never see our bodies as they are from the perspective of our own body. As he says: "But when it comes to my body, I never observe it itself. I would need a second body to be able to do so, which would itself be unobservable" (Merleau-Ponty, 1945, p. 95). Both Sartre and Merleau-Ponty recognised that the body exists on two distinct levels in relation to consciousness: that of the 'in-itself' and the 'for-itself'—the 'in itself' relating to the felt and affective dimension of physical experience and the 'for-itself' pertaining to the object status of the body within the field and realm of appearances.

In our modern times, as shifts occur in religious beliefs and in the role of the Other (as the guarantor of meaning) within ideology, understandings of subjectivity become more focused on internal factors rather than on external ones (such as God). In many disciplines, including science, psychoanalysis, and fields such as feminism, theatre studies, and disability studies, attempts have been made to situate the body as more central to the experience of the individual, although there is a difference in what is considered to be the body in these debates. In psychoanalytic theory, for example, the body is not reducible to the organism, being in part a construct of language, and in science, the body is often aligned with the brain, or the brain with the mind, rather than being seen as a discursive entity.

### *Defining the Gap*

In some ways, privileging the body as central to the experience of the human subject has led paradoxically (in response to the purported Cartesian mind/body split) to a collapse in the distinction or gap between body and mind, minimising the reality of the fragility of the body and the nature of contingencies that surround embodiment. Descartes' reasoning has influenced conceptualisations of a binary being, split between body and mind, in which the rationality of thought takes precedence over the fleshy materiality of the body. His (in)famous statement of *cogito ergo sum*, 'I think therefore I am,' places the ego or the one who is thinking as central to the ontological question of existence and centres doubt as a marker of existence. However, as we have already seen, Galadí (2023) critiques Descartes' position as being a hidden one of ontological identification with the mental realm: 'I am what I think'. In other words, Descartes doesn't know he has made this identification of mind with being. In a reversal of this identification, Lacan's teachings on the divided subject completely and deliberately undercut Descartes's privileging of the 'I' as central to the experience of knowledge and instead, the unconscious becomes the locus of the subject's decentralisation and of being. For example, in *Seminar IX, Identification*, Lacan argues against Descartes's proposal that thinking proves the existence of the subject:

> 'I think' is not a thought. Descartes, of course, proposes these formulae at the end of a long process of thinking, and it is quite certain that the thinking involved is the thinking of a thinker. I would go even further: this characteristic, it is a thinking of a thinker, is not required for us to talk about thought. A thought, in a word, in no way requires that one thinks about the thought. For us in particular, thinking begins with the unconscious.
>
> (Lacan, Lesson 1, 15 November 1961–1962, p. 7)

To state that thinking begins with the unconscious is something of a conundrum, as it brings into question the nature of representation in the unconscious and at what level we think and how, given, as Cox Cameron (2026, forthcoming publication) points out in a study seminar on *Seminar IX Identification*, language is not directly a feature of the unconscious, though the unconscious may be structured like a language. Aside from determining the register of thinking, the other point being made here is that the 'I' or the thinker of Cartesian thought is not the same thinker of the thoughts of the Lacanian unconscious. Unconscious thinking, as I understand it, happens without the control of the personal pronoun or the 'I' of the statement. Given Descartes' emphasis on the certainty of the thinker's position as proof of existence, and its opposition to the substance of the body, the philosopher is often attributed with influencing binary paradigms of thought regarding body/mind. As Dunne and Butler point out, such paradigms "legitimize a patriarchal and phallocentric mode of reasoning" (2012, p. 1). Furthermore, this phallocentric mode of reasoning privileges a binary view of gender, where rationality is favoured over the 'emotional or leaky body' and hence masculinity over femininity, given that rationality is often associated with the male of the species and the emotional with the female. However, as Harrington (2008) points out, and my intuition agrees, the cultural attribution and emphasis placed on Descartes regarding the mind–body split symbolise a nostalgia for a time when mind and body seemingly enjoyed a mythical harmony of oneness.

So, while Descartes's cogito symbolises a theoretical divide between body and mind, at the other end of the mind–body duality debate lie equally erroneous conceptions (tacit or overt) that privilege a harmonious, symmetrical mind-body unity—think of the cult of positive thinking and how the body can be healed through positive affirmations. It could be said that there is a gap in knowledge concerning the gap that appears to exist in the relationship between body and mind, or in our explanation of this relationship. Even today, the epistemological gap concerning this connection remains a stubborn, unresolved issue. Furthermore, attempts to fill this gap in the nature of psyche and soma have led to problematic, overdetermined interpretations of bodily or psychic events. This can be seen in the increasing popularity of employing various psychological practices, such as cognitive behavioural therapy, as interventions for disease and illness in the medical field. Although a holistic approach is laudable and there are always psychological issues to be dealt with concerning illness, it is the overarching way these therapies are utilised that speaks of somatically orientated theoretical simplifications. Of course, it really depends on the degree of emphasis with which these interventions are employed and on the qualitative evaluation of effectiveness, i.e. whether they are aimed at cure vs quality-of-life modifications. In "Subject and Body" (2001), Paul Verhaeghe, in his study of the theorisation of the body across decades of Lacan's work, notes that attempts to suture the gap between psyche and soma have further reinforced it, as these attempts fail to understand what distinguishes the gap in the first place. In contrast to this misplaced suturing, which, at its core, rests on a binary understanding of psyche and soma, he argues that the trajectory of Lacan's thought concerning the body, from the early to the later seminars, offers a new way of thinking through the connections between the subject and the body. As Verhaeghe writes:

> If we study Lacan's entire work, we find a more complex relationship between the subject and the body, one that differs from the classical opposition between psyche and soma. The Lacanian opposition is between the I and the body as an organism and this leads to an opposition between the divided subject and the sexualised, that is, phallicised body.
>
> (Verhaeghe, 2001, p. 18)

Notwithstanding the complexity of this statement and the puzzling opposition of a sexualised and phallicised body, this account of the division between the 'I' and the body as an organism contextualises the split inherent to subjectivity as more than simply dual, and highlights the problematic nature of the traditional mind–body debate that analyses a relationship in terms of a binary. For Lacan, the body is not a whole entity, something that can be completed or sutured, but rather is composed of 'holes' (Brenner, 2021). These holes concern the incompleteness of meaning inherent to the interacting registers of the Real, the imaginary, and the symbolic. Through his reading of the trajectory of the theorisation of the body, and its transition from the body of the symbolic to the body of the Real, Verhaeghe argues that "the human subject is not a divided subject but a quartered being" (2001, p. 21). In this quaternary understanding of the subject, divided into several levels of subjectivity, where the attempt to fill one lack only highlights another, we move away from the polarities of separation and unity inherent to the concepts of mind and body, or even splitting, into a more complex terrain of topological ambiguity. We must keep in mind that what differentiates the theory of the body in psychoanalysis from other academic, philosophical, or literary domains is the presence of the unconscious within the theoretical and clinical paradigm and the fact that the subject of the unconscious is not the same subject as the I who speaks—although we could say it is spoken by, or infused by, this unconscious subject. While identifying the unconscious as central to the debate on the body, this present study also needs to tailor this approach to the specifics of reading the body in theatre. We will see, however, in the next chapters, that working with the unconscious in the artistic context is not easy and involves a certain leap of faith—a belief in its existence. It is not something that can be measured or proven empirically, although many clinicians who have worked with the unconscious in the consulting room might differ about that view. Nonetheless, in any psychoanalytic account of the body, we must be critically aware of the role of the unconscious, either in the construction of a body or in the description of our lived experience.

### *The Unconscious Disrupts the Binary*

In psychoanalysis, the unconscious is privileged as central to existence and in contrast to ideals of harmony, introduces a discontinuity, an Otherness within subjectivity. Although existing within us to a degree, the unconscious is a dimension of Otherness, and its presence subverts any coherent or stable sense of identity that could be imagined to be a core originality of being. Subjectivity is, as Lacan says, "always a question of the subject qua indeterminate" (Lacan, 1964/1978, p. 26). As the realm of the indeterminate, the unconscious serves as a mediating point between the organic matter of the body and the symbolic structures of self-identity. This mediation of the unconscious is facilitated and expressed by processes of representation concerning language and other signifiers. By taking account of the position of the unconscious in embodied subjectivity, we can broaden the previous debates on the mind/body problem. No longer do we have to remain within a binary model where mind and body are conceived as separate substances or, at the other extreme, as a union of symmetrical proportion. Instead, we can conceptualise the issue as being neither one nor the other, but as something infinitely more complex. As Lacan argues in a critique of phenomenological thinking regarding mind/body dualism:

> This path, which is rich with a whole cornucopia of facts, affords us something that for a long time has struck us as very desirable, namely, the solution of mind/body dualism. It sees the body, taken at the functional level, as a kind of double, the lining, of all the functions of the mind. We should not be satisfied with this, however, because there is still some sleight of hand going on.
>
> (Lacan, 2014, p. 219)

This sleight of hand, as Lacan puts it, is because the body and mind cannot be conceived of as a closed system, a set of all sets, or even as two distinct entities, but rather as a dynamic of multiple registers that do not add up neatly to a singular unit. This lack of unity relates to the concept of the object a as that marker of an 'object' that is lost to the body and that can never be recovered. If we take as a premise for our argument that the body and mind are not one whole, nor are they separate, as in there is no mind without a body, where does that leave us with the definition of the body we set out to determine in this chapter? And how will it help us in the elaborations that follow? I contend it is the very slipperiness of this answer and its perplexing complexity that is at the heart of problematic mind–body narratives, narratives that we will see in the next chapter work to underpin idealisations of the self and subjectivity while ultimately deriding or invalidating less ideal realities, such as that of corporeal difference or alternate modalities of being and doing. For example, social discourse tends to privilege narratives or stories where the mind appears to be a great strength and source of power, the conveyor of a strong will, and where it has the capacity to drive the body into achieving or performing impressive tasks, such as being an Olympian runner or the CEO of a billion-dollar enterprise. Therefore, the idea that the mind can control and manifest desired 'successful' scenarios is one such problematic narrative, for while it may be true in some instances, it also perpetuates the category of the neoliberal able-bodied subject who only has to put their 'mind' to something to achieve it. This narrative of mind over matter, or what Harrington (2008) calls the narrative of positive thinking, is deeply ingrained in our culture, and one of the difficulties in critiquing it is that the mind does indeed have a great influence on the body, but not always. The theoretical underpinning of this narrative of overcoming is, I argue, that the mind and body are one, or at least reciprocal, and that what the mind thinks consciously, the body can do. While this may be true sometimes, it is clearly not the case in many scenarios. This ambiguity is the critical caveat. We must remember that, psychoanalytically, conscious thinking is bracketed as not being the voice of authority over our being, and we can be wary whenever something seems to be consciously wished for or desired, of the potential for short-circuiting by unconscious means. Ultimately I argue that the reason the question of the body is so difficult to answer is that it belies a trauma, a hole in knowledge concerning cause. That this aspect of the body cannot be known renders it a form of trauma.

The issue of substance versus interpretation, the fact that perception is of critical importance to the experience and definition of embodiment as well as biological materiality, does not erode the contingent properties of the flesh as a material traumatic substance. In fact, this is one of the paradoxes of embodiment: perception, fantasy, and the imaginary all determine our experience of the body, yet, in my view, there is nonetheless a materiality at work that produces psychic or emotional effects that are hard to determine. Similarly, ambiguities abound when attempting to localise or anchor the body within subjectivity; this aspect concerns the very nature of human beings reflecting on the composition of their own bodies. We understand things through the dimension of the signifier; language distorts and causes splitting within the objects of our study, lending a certain porousness to the narratives that form to shield us from the abyssal dimensions of embodiment.

## Note

1 For a comprehensive and accessible discussion of the question of what the mind is and its epistemological parameters, see Mark Solms (2015). Interestingly, from the perspective of knowledge in this book, the mind, according to Solms, is unknowable directly and yet it can be inferred and experienced through perception. As he puts it: "The mind in itself, like all ultimate things, can only be modelled; it cannot be observed directly."

## References

Berger, J. (2004). Trauma without disability, disability without trauma: A disciplinary divide. *JAC Special Issue, Part 2: Trauma and Rhetoric, 24(3)*, 563–582.

Brenner, L. (2021). Is the autistic body a body without organs? In B. McLaughlin & E. Daffron (Eds.) *The body in theory: Essays after Lacan and Foucault*. pp. 42–56. McFarland & Company.

Butler, N. & Dunne, S. (2012). Duelling with dualisms: Descartes, Foucault and the history of organizational limits. *Management and Organisational History*, 7 (12).

Cox Cameron, O. (2026). *Studying Seminar IX*. study seminar (edited by Carol Owens and Sarah Meehan O'Callaghan) forthcoming. Routledge.

Freud, S. (1915). Instincts and their vicissitudes (J. Strachey, Transl.). In *The standard edition of the complete psychological works of Sigmund Freud, Volume XIV (1914–1916)*. London: Hogarth Press.
Freud, S. (1917). Mourning and melancholia. In *The standard edition of the complete psychological works of Sigmund Freud, Volume XIV (1914–1916): On the history of the psycho-analytic movement, papers on metapsychology and other works*. London: Vintage.
Freud, S. (1923). The Ego and the Id. *In The standard edition of the complete psychological works of Sigmund Freud, Volume XIX (1923–1925): The Ego and the Id and Other Works*. 1–66.
Galadí J. A (2023). What I am and what I am not: *Destruktion* of the mind–body problem. *Philosophies* 8, 110. doi:10.3390/philosophies8060110
Harrington, A. (2008). *The cure within: A history of mind-body medicine*. New York & London: Norton.
Lacan, J. (1961–62). *The seminar of Jacques Lacan: Seminar IX Identification*. (C. Gallagher, Transl.) Unpublished.
Lacan, J. (1964/1978). *The seminar of Jacques Lacan. The four fundamental concepts of psychoanalysis*. (J. A. Miller, Ed., & A. Sheridan, Transl.) New York: Norton.
Lacan, J. (1976–1977). *L'insu que sait. Seminar XXIV. Final sessions*. (C. Gallagher, Transl.) Unpublished.
Lacan, J. (2014). *Anxiety: The seminar of Jacques Lacan, Book X*. (J.-A. Miller, Ed.; A. R. Price, Trans.). Polity.
Merleau-Ponty. (1944). *Phenomenology of perception*. Routledge.
Soler, C. (1984). The body in the teaching of Lacan. https://jcfar.org.uk/wp-content/uploads/2016/03/The-Body-in-the-Teaching-of-Jacques-Lacan-Colette-Soler.pdf.
Solms, M. (2015). *The feeling brain. Selected papers on neuropsychoanalysis*. Kamac.
Solms, M. (2019). The hard problem of consciousness and the free energy principle. *Frontiers in Psychology*. 9, 2714.
Verhaeghe, P. (2001). Subject and body. Lacan's struggle with the real. In P. Verhaeghe, *Beyond gender: from subject to drive* (pp. 65–97). New York: Other Press.

Chapter 2

# The Problem with Mind–Body Narratives

Human beings reside in a world of storytelling, myths, belief systems, and narratives. In modern times, how we understand our existence is a product of scientific discovery and the influence of an underlying network of transgenerational philosophical and religious ideas. As we have seen, the conception of a body and the terms of debate over the 'problem' of the body–mind connection are products of narratives embedded in a long historical pursuit of investigation and philosophical speculation. Extending this context, this chapter centres on the human being as a subject of narrative, with a particular focus on how cultural, social, and discipline-specific narratives—while essential components of existence and intrinsic features of inter- and intra-personal relationships—can have problematic and stigmatising effects. While the question of the body is fundamentally ontological and indefinable, narratives can be understood as responses to the enigma it poses. Firstly, what is a mind–body narrative?

## The Narrative of Ableism

In short, problematic mind–body narratives are stories or paradigms of the body–mind connection around which complex truths/realities/experiences of the body or mind are obscured in favour of simpler understandings of what constitutes a body/mind or the relation between them. I will focus in particular on the concept of ableism, which in essence is a prejudice against disability and an idealisation of so-called productive bodies, as a source of problematic narratives that place the mind (or what is construed as the mind) as the predominant agent of selfhood and differential states of embodiment as inferior to conceptions of the self as whole, autonomous, rational, and able. The narratives within which ableism can be traced are varied and pervasive, historical and contemporary, and operate not simply to stigmatise physical disability but also psychiatric or mental conditions—think of the sterilisation of people with mental illness in the last century and the extermination of those with physical or mental disabilities by the Nazis. While these examples are extreme, they occurred as a result of ideas or narratives about what was believed to be the optimal and desirable level of functioning

DOI: 10.4324/9781003509622-4

for a human being. While narrative per se is not a bad thing, and is probably an essential modality for humans to organise and make sense of experience, the ones under discussion here are problematic not simply because they shield us from more difficult realisations at the level of truth, but because they can impact on anything from the quality of interpersonal relationships to the provision of social resources and effective medical care.

Mind–body narratives find their way into all aspects of life, from the throwaway remarks someone might make to a person with cancer about looking well despite their illness (the underlying assumption being that being ill must make you look sick and wellness is about appearance) to the ideological tenets underlying neoliberal conceptualisations of the productive subject (we can be autonomous and achieve anything we put our mind to, the body will follow). Therefore there is no situation that is impossible to overcome; it is just a question of attitude and focus. There are narratives within psychiatry that concern the biological cause of mental illness and its related treatment with drugs, in which the brain is purported (without adequate evidence to date, see Harrington 2019) to be the cause of numerous mental disorders and there are narratives that centre on the mind causing somatic illness or functional neurological disorder (again often without adequate evidence). There are narratives within psychoanalysis concerning hysteria and conversion disorder. Even I would say that any explanation that becomes wholesale for theories of the construction of the self, such as the alienated, split, and divided subject of the unconscious, is a narrative. Effectively narratives provide us with a shared lexicon to access paradigms of thought or cultivate belief systems. They are signifiers that repeat and provide subjects with narcissistic stability within a discourse. We can think of Lacan's concept of a master signifier, S1, here, the S1 being the nonsensical signifier that nonetheless grounds a discourse, within which the S2s circulate as knowledge production. The S1 is the shorthand for the main idea or belief that supports the narrative around which the other signifiers form a social link based on a presumption of knowledge. It is difficult to say how cultural narratives form, as there are so many layers involved, but perhaps we can understand one aspect by thinking of the human being's need to attribute meaning and order to experience and the need to infer causality to events, even where the actual causality might be contingent or chance-related (Kahneman, 2011). To understand and contextualise why something might have happened, we recount events and tell stories, and live our lives through portals of fiction, where the boundaries between fact and narrated story often blur. From a psychoanalytic point of view, of course, fiction is not simply make-believe but integral to the very conditions of our linguistically-structured symbolic networks. As subjects of language, we are born of fictions and will probably die within their grasp; nonetheless, we can be aware of the temptation to imagine causes for intractable dilemmas, and how this may manifest at a cultural level.

Keeping in mind this tendency of the human subject to apply meaning and signification to the enigmas of the world around them and to seek simplified answers to complex problems, I propose that narratives form threads of meaning within the broader spheres of discourse across many fields and disciplines. They are modes of comprehending the often incomprehensible, of grouping and organising, or coagulating many different factors and disparate fragments of a debate into an overarching, coherent story. For example, the notion of trauma as an occurrence that engenders an experience outside representation has become a very common and popular hermeneutic trope in therapeutic and academic spheres. Effectively, trauma, that signifier of deep distress and unknowability, has become a narrative, a way of understanding hidden, incomprehensible, and troubled realms of the self, a culturally predominant story of being in the modern world. Narratives are interwoven into discourse as stories or conventional belief systems, tacit or overt, that seem to provide answers to complex problems. Narratives are not untruths per se; rather, they take individual facts and singular truths and make them collective and comprehensive. For example, facts and observed clinical phenomena of certain bodies in distress, certain suffering minds, may become narratives in the sense of one-size-fits-all approaches to therapeutic care—just think of the pervasive prescriptions for antidepressants. These narratives may include the idea that the body stores traumatic experiences, and sometimes, depending on the therapeutic orientation, the idea that trauma can be released through bodywork; a view that differs from, for example, Lacanian psychoanalysis, where the emphasis is on speech and the signifier. The difference, I would say here, is that from a Lacanian point of view, trauma is not something to be healed categorically, and so releasing it from the body would be an endless process. And yet, we must be careful in this putative differentiation as speech is an embodied activity, and language, from a Lacanian point of view, traumatises the body and is written upon it; therefore, speaking (in the presence of another) *is* a form of bodywork, as the body is implicated within the speech we utter as enunciator and the speech we receive from the other. As Colette Soler (1984) points out, psychoanalysis may be a form of physical therapy. These narratives concerning the relationship between body and mind are not new, although they may take different forms. Indeed, as Anne Harrington (2008) shows in *The Cure Within,* current narratives or beliefs surrounding contemporary paradigms of mind–body medicine often have their roots in historically relevant discourses, such as the influence of religion on medicine and the idea of confessing sins as an antidote to damnation and illness. Generally, without concrete evidence to explain the cause of a phenomenon, human beings are subject to speculation and attempt to find meaning in mystery; furthermore, not only is meaning found in mystery, but mystery is actively sought out, for when we do find scientific answers, these are not always satisfactory.

Nowhere can this be truer than in the history of speculation and theory concerning the mind–body connection. Although the resonance of the age-old Cartesian debate concerning the relationship of body and mind, psyche and soma is implicit in the category of mind–body narratives and the very construction of the terminology, the way this relationship manifests is polyvalent. In other words, whether the mind and body are one entity (monism) or separate entities (dualism) that cannot be collapsed into the same substance is one route for exploring the narratives that subtend our existence in many ways. Certainly, these broader paradigms conjure narratives, either macro or micro, in themselves, the most prevalent being that the mind and body are a mutually reflecting unit, an indivisible system of reciprocal exchange. The consequence of this view, in its most extreme form, is that we may be able to think our way out of a dilemma through positive thinking (e.g., the view of Louise Hay or the populist advice given by healing and health gurus). However, this type of thinking is also a byproduct of less obviously bifurcated narratives circulating in our socio-cultural-political realm. That is, beneath the tropes and idealisations of socio-cultural discourse may lie simplifications of what constitutes the body and its relation to the psyche in the first place. That these simplifications are hidden through populist rhetoric is a function of the tendency of the human being to economise and take shortcuts in cognitive comprehension. This idea has been illustrated by a number of thinkers across different disciplines; for example, the empirical orientation of Dan Kahneman in *Thinking, Fast and Slow* and his discussion of how much thinking and cognition are embodied activities that require significant brain effort. From the perspective of neuroscience, in his quest to discover the truth of consciousness, Antonio Damasio (1999) describes how the body can be hidden or veiled by the mind as a form of adaptation to the external world:

> Sometimes we use our minds to hide a part of our beings from another part of our beings. I could describe the hiding of the body as a distraction, but I would have to add that it is a very adaptive distraction. In most circumstances, rather than concentrating resources on our inner states, it is perhaps more advantageous to concentrate one's resources on the images that describe problems out in the world or on the premises of those problems or on the options for their solution and their possible outcomes. Yet this skewing of perspective relative to what is available in our minds has a cost. It tends to prevent us from sensing the possible origin and nature of what we call self.

Or, as Dan Collins reminds us (forthcoming publication 2026) in a reading of Lacan's *Seminar IX, Identification* and Lacan's request for the reader to think, thinking is not easy, and certainly, thinking that steps outside the imaginary domain of everyday language and familiar representation systems may be rarely done. Even if such thinking is conducted, it is not easy to convey in a language that is transmissible, as Lacan's lucubrations through topological shapes are testament to. Similarly, *in Why do People Get Ill? Exploring the Mind–Body Connection*, Darian Leader points out the tendency, regarding understanding the somewhat enigmatic relationship between body and mind in illness, to seek simplified answers to complicated situations. He gives the example of the purported single cause theory of biological illness as an example of how neat theories of singular causality can satisfy the desire to know, treat medically, account for, or attribute meaning to an event, as in the case of the bacteria that was found to be a causative factor in ulcers. Leader opens the terms of the debate to include the wider context of symbolic and unconscious factors involved in people becoming ill, but does not mention the harm that these more psychological ideas can also have on those living with disability or chronic illness. Although I use psychoanalysis in this book to interrogate mind–body narratives through the work of Beckett and Artaud, I also wish to challenge it regarding its own purchase on what I feel are its ableist-inflected assumptions about agency, productivity, and corporeality.

The rest of this chapter briefly discusses the ramifications and associated narratives of ableism. In short, ableism is the privileging of bodies that are apparently functioning and 'able' to perform certain tasks over bodies that may be impaired and lacking in functionality or diminished productive capacity. This privileging of functionality finds its way into all sorts of judgements and presumptions about how a person lives or their lifestyle. It is not strictly limited to judgments on the body per se, as in the stigma of appearing physically different or being obviously restricted in some way, but also occurs in what might be considered the realm of the mind—the forever tricky distinction—examples being judgements around ambition, career choice, degree of activity, etc. In fact, there are a multitude of examples in which the reason behind career choice, employment, or even family configuration may be a physical one but this is not comprehensible to the person outside this situation. We tend to infer psychic causality to physical phenomena, sometimes for good reason but also fallaciously.

We should keep in mind that historically, and still in some respects to this day, disability was seen as a moral failing (Goodley, 2011). Hence, an impairment, ailment, or limitation of the body was understood to be the reflection of some sort of sin or sickness within the mind or soul of an individual. Of course, in earlier centuries, we did not have the benefit of science to explain the cause of many diseases (though actual cause rather than measurable symptomology can still be very much disputed), so in a sense, humans relied more on myth and meaning to make sense of the unexplainable, and religion with its ready-made meaning system was a helpful fallback in times of crisis. To see a physical ailment as a manifestation of sin was, in essence, placing the failing of the body somehow as the fault of the individual. This perspective was not too dissimilar from how narratives of the body expressing a hidden truth have circulated around the concept of hysteria. The genesis of hysteria in the nineteenth century, its development by Freud, and the understanding that repressed psychic material can manifest through physiological symptoms led to the well-known aphorism within psychoanalytic/psychotherapy circles that 'the body speaks.' Indeed, this is one of the six key historical mind-body narratives identified by Harrington (2008) that permeate our present-day culture in altered forms. In this narrative, the body expresses the mind's discontent, particularly when something is not spoken, and serves as a 'writing pad' for unconscious conflicts. The actual mechanisms by which the body translates mental or unconscious stimuli (such as thoughts) into physical symptoms or disorders seem hard to pinpoint. Speculations are often enigmatic, involving the complex interplay of affects, thoughts, symbolism, physiological processes, and maybe multiple registers of mind. It is worth noting, according to the Neuropsychoanalytic Association, that hysteria or conversion disorder is now referred to in contemporary medicine as functional neurological disorder, with functional implying a lack of knowledge about the aetiology of the condition or an assumption that the condition borders the psychiatric domain.

## The Narrative of Conversion Disorder

A great deal of research is currently being conducted at the intersections of the brain, mind, and body, yet historical mind–body narratives remain alive and well. For example, the 2024 Neuropsychoanalytic Congress focused on "When the Body Speaks: Conversion Disorder and Beyond" underscored the topic's continued relevance today. While I'm not disputing the validity of this taxonomy, I think it is important to recognise that the insights of Freud often become converted into simplifications and shorthand that can end up stigmatising people with physiological conditions or disabilities. Admittedly, the juxtaposition of the topic of disability with that of hysteria is somewhat tenuous, as we have the ambiguous question of what exactly constitutes a disability, let alone hysteria, but nonetheless, making a connection between these fields is relevant in understanding prevailing attitudes towards disabilities or illnesses of unknown origin, particularly in the medical field. This conceptual conflation is a factor in the prevalence of gaslighting, which exists wholesale across countries and continents in relation to diseases, illnesses, or physiological states that confound scientific knowledge. While functional neurological disorder may be a valid taxonomy, the fallout of these nominations for people with 'undocumented illness' or poorly understood complex disorders that, through a certain paucity of diagnosis, fall within the functional category, is rarely acknowledged in psychoanalysis. This is one of the features of ableism: in essence, a blindness to the impact of theories and practices that marginalise or further alienate differential bodies and experiences, or, we could even say, deviant bodies. It is important to note that those who may fall into the categories of deviant, less functional, differentially embodied, or non-average can also develop or perpetuate problematic narratives about the mind–body connection, either in the singular or in group form. My point here is to highlight the pervasiveness of the human tendency to be seduced into creating stories and finding causality in meaning-laced accounts that, although possibly structured around aspects of truth, overshoot and lie somewhere on the shores of individual and collective fantasy.

By way of extrapolating what is problematic about certain mind–body narratives, I will begin with an anecdote taken from my own life. A number of years ago, I was attending a neuropsychoanalytic conference, and a speaker (a neurologist) was elaborating on a case of functional neurological disorder by way of a video and a description of the case. The video presented footage of a patient who was suffering from a version of psychic Parkinson's disease or some similar neurological condition, and this condition, albeit somewhat apparently imagined, affected their gait and movement. As it was a functional disorder, the implication was that this was not a real bodily disorder, a problem with the organic body, but one that originated in the mind. That this illness was somewhat imaginary was also underlined by the chorus of laughter emanating from the audience. It seemed that the group of clinicians found it funny to witness someone who did not *really* have Parkinson's but only thought they had. The stinging laughter of a crowd of clinicians about the fate of a patient who may traditionally have been described as suffering from hysteria serves to underline the attitudes of ableism and the stigma affecting many people with disabilities, both within and outside the psychoanalytic community. So what was the laughter about, we may ask? Although I can't be definitive, it very much seemed that the butt of the joke was the seemingly imagined nature of the condition and the ridiculousness of walking with an altered gait, which was not caused by any real physiological cause. I am firmly of the belief that attitudes towards medically unexplained illness often take the form of derision and rely on presumptions of inferior self-awareness. Anna Mollow (2018) has referred to this attitude as pertaining to the question of knowledge in undocumented illness, where people with these disabilities are seen as epistemologically disabled; that is, there is something of themselves they do not know that has caused their physical illness or disability, and they are somehow in an inferior position to the able-bodied person who has not fallen victim to this epistemological trap. Within this category of the epistemologically disabled fall narratives of trauma, or the presumption that the person who is ill may not have dealt with trauma. So, in other words, perhaps the audience laughed from a position of superiority at the presentation of the patient's state of 'unknowability' toward them. The patient's seeming blindness to their own lack of knowledge was a source of amusement.

And so what can be learned about body–mind narratives from this anecdote? I think the answer lies in an examination of the roots of ableism, an outlook on life blinkered by the perspective of able-bodiedness and the normative modes of production, its place within psychoanalysis, and the beliefs or narratives surrounding the body–mind connection that underlie its manifestation. In an article on the distinctions between racism and ableism in psychoanalysis, the late Christina Emanuel, speaking from a perspective influenced by post-colonial theory and the incendiary language of Fanon, states that psychoanalysis needs to be blown apart to recognise its own prejudice or bias in this area and to recognise disability or bodily difference as one of the manifestations of difference and factors of oppression affecting clients, along with race, class, sexuality, and potentially themselves: "I believe that when it comes to redressing the ignorance of unanalysed ableism and disability, psychoanalysis indeed needs to be blown apart too" (Emanuel, 2022).

Indeed, when it comes to disability studies, psychoanalysis is not a favoured theoretical model (Shildrick (2009), Anna Mollow (2018)) with which to analyse the modes of stigma and oppression pertaining to differential embodiment within the sociocultural domain or with which to interrogate the experience of the disabled subject. This is in part because psychoanalysis, given its clinical focus, is viewed as pathologising or medicalising the experience of ontologically alternate subjects without offering alternate models of becoming, unlike, as Shildrick (2009) argues, Deleuzian theory, which proposes such models. Another reason why psychoanalysis may not be popular within disability studies is the lack of literature on this topic within the psychoanalytic canon; there are so few references and studies to work with. By contrast, psychoanalysis does feature as a theoretical paradigm within disability studies, although sparingly and with some stated reservations by scholars in the field, such as Goodley (2011). The association of psychoanalysis with psychic pathology (and concepts such as secondary gain from illness) have been discouraging for theorists attempting to break free of medical models of disability (where the individual is othered as being deficient) or who feel a psychoanalytic emphasis on the subject (as in the Lacanian sense) of disability takes away from political debates and the dismantling of oppression within societal hierarchies. It's interesting how prominent the presence of the body is in psychoanalysis, yet generally, theory tends to surround the psyche's role in bodily symptomatology and not the other way round. Could this lack of focus on disability in psychoanalysis be related to a resistance to the fact that, as Emanuel points out, disability is something that has the potential to affect everybody, given the adage that at some point in their lives, all people will experience a restriction of movement through ageing, accident, or disease, and thus in this way disability is unlike, for example, race? And yet, the topic of the non-normative body or the disabled body should also be a question for the consulting room and for the praxis of psychoanalysis.

I argue that a deeper, and possibly novel, engagement with the ideas of Lacan and Freud than one usually finds in disability-orientated theory can open other avenues for conceiving differences within psychoanalysis, including highlighting the very immanent differences that subjects have within themselves. Similarly, disability studies can benefit from psychoanalytic thinking, as I hold that what is lacking within disability studies is an exploration of the divided subject as singular and as being, just like non-disabled people, subject to what I argue is the ontological trauma of the body. In some senses, then, there is an ableism at work within some narratives[1] of disability communities and fields of study, an ableism that denies the inherent splitness of the subject of the unconscious or that denies the unconscious as being a feature of disability or physical difference. From a psychoanalytic perspective, it is clear that all bodies are subject to traumas and enjoyments (plural), which does not mean that all bodies are technically disabled as a result, but rather that there is no stable point of enduring body–mind identification; it, or at least its ego-related aspect, can be disrupted at any time. I find Freud's (1923) definition of the ego as "first and foremost a body-ego" (p. 26), an entity derived from internal bodily sensations,[2] helpful in understanding the implications of changes to the physical body, including the body's role in identification and the potential collapse the subject may experience at this level. I wonder if this inherent precarity of the subject of the body is one of the reasons disability studies tends to avoid the concept of trauma, as there is a tendency to want to highlight autonomy and bodily integrity over stigmatising and pejorative views of dependence and powerlessness. Yet, in my view, this is another avenue of ableism, the erroneous belief in mastery and the denial of the lack at the heart of embodied being, that which concerns the impossibility of a full knowledge of ourselves at any given time and the vulnerable underside of culturally-ideal ego identifications, identifications that often privilege action-orientated movements or, to put it simply, doing over being.

## Narratives of Being, Doing, and the Will

Ableism is more than a negative appraisal of being different. Often, it involves a completely different worldview that seems impossible for some non-disabled people to imagine without resorting to the dictates of positive thinking or the idea of an autonomous self-improving will. In other words, as Josh Cohen (2019) points out regarding the culture of overactivity and the unrelenting capitalist pace of our twenty-first-century world in *Not Working: Why We Have to Stop*, working and the pursuit of action are valued over being or doing nothing. Underlying this frenetic activity is a belief in the ideal (Cohen refers to the ego-ideal) that anything is possible; we can be anything we want to be, it is simply our attitude that fails us. While psychoanalysis is perfectly positioned to critique this idea from the perspective of the unconscious and non-rational self—as in the work of Paul Verhaeghe (2014) concerning the idealism of the self and neoliberalism, not to mention

Lacan's idea that being and thought are oppositional: "I am where I do not think" (Lacan, 2006, p. 430)—I think, ironically, that this view is also to an extent an unconscious undercurrent in psychoanalysis, as psychoanalysts and psychoanalytic scholars are not immune to the effects of the societal brainwashing of our contemporary times, even if we are critiquing and aware of them. This is an important paradox to underline and reflect on. We can theorise, write, and practise from the perspective of Lacanian or whatever clinical or theoretical orientation we may take up, but that does not mean we are not subject to veils of ignorance, or at least flashes of ignorance concerning bias, and are not impelled towards the seductions of social conformism. It is not easy to pursue or be true to our desire and forsake the realm of the goods (Meehan O'Callaghan, 2024) when we are subjects who live in society and may suffer consequences for being true to that desire by, for example, standing up to a militant regime or standing out from the crowd in some way that goes against the status quo. Nor is it easy to challenge the ableist rhetoric of doing and becoming someone over being (no one).

The rhetoric of doing over being contains a view on the nature of volition and the body or what we could also call the will and organic matter. Although of course the body as organic matter is debatable, let us consider the issue at hand in attitudes towards what the body can or cannot do in the normative sense (and possibly the neoliberal sense of body as action, as agent of productivity, as signifier of the labour required toward the fulfilment of some end). Regarding ableism, aside from the myriad of potential discriminatory markers pertaining to disability, such as the stigma of physical difference, and the socio-economic consequences of certain conditions, I argue we are fundamentally dealing with a reaction to states of doing or not doing, movement and stasis, and a denial of the underlying state of the human as being or non-being. Again, Josh Cohen's arguments concerning the prejudice against doing nothing and states of sloth, lassitude, laziness, and daydreaming as avenues to experience a less frenetic type of being are pertinent here. He explains that there is a societal aversion to these states because, at some level, this drive towards doing nothing is within us all, and so this desire for non-desire is projected onto those accused of being slackers or welfare cheats, etc. By saying that, I do not mean to imply that people with disabilities do not do things, but I am looking at it through a particular lens in which certain physical conditions lead to a state of diminished doing. In these situations, action is greatly reduced, restricted, or slowed much more than average. I am conscious of the challenge Goodley (2011) makes regarding the responsibility of a writer or researcher in the field of disability towards advancing equality and not perpetuating stigma through erroneous stereotyping and misplaced psychologisation. Nonetheless, I think it is critically important to recognise certain realities and frustrations within states of impairment, which are not necessarily alleviated by a post-structural linguistic deconstruction of the hierarchical import of binary oppositions in cultural discursive categories, such as male/female, sex/gender, able/disabled. The aim here is more epistemological rather than activist in that I am interested in how narratives of the body–mind connection also surface problematically within disability studies or how disability studies may fall prey to simplifications concerning the body—accounts of the body that do not take into account the unconscious and the divided subject, for example. How is disability or physical suffering lived at the visceral level, at the level of sensation and its psychic correlations or representations? Many disabilities do not involve specific issues of movement, but many do, and, if we look closely, maybe more than would first appear, and these are the ones I know most about. For example, somebody with a visual impairment will have difficulty moving around, not because of an issue with functional movement, but because it is hard to navigate the environment without sight. In these situations, we need to think about movement differently than when we do it automatically, so it becomes present to our consciousness.

And yet what causes us to move? Is it our thoughts and our will or something else? Is it a tension at the level of the body? It may be the case that, like Heidegger's hammer, which, when working properly, is not deconstructed as an object, we are only aware of bodily movements, at least in acute detail, when it becomes difficult to make them. If we think about it, we may assume that we intend our movements—that is, we instruct our body or mind to do things according to what we imagine, desire, or cultivate in our mind's eye. If we consider the most basic action we can do to get up from a chair and make a cup of tea, we need a certain amount of volition and will to motivate and move ourselves into action. Or do we? Is it will, or is it something else? Are we intending, or are we being intended? When are we impelled by need, such as hunger or thirst, and when by desire (to distinguish between the excessive dimension of desire as that which exceeds need)? At a later point, I will more closely examine this idea of volition and the body through Beckett's works and, according to Rabaté, his favourite philosopher Geulincx[3] (2016, p. 45), whose philosophy of occasionalism purports that our actions are caused by something which we cannot know, so we are moved but it is not really our will moving us; we cannot really say how we moved, and we don't have full knowledge of it.

As we shall see, the trope of moving and not moving is hugely significant throughout Beckett's oeuvre as the stage directions of *Waiting for Godot* illustrate:

> Vladimir: "Well, shall we go?"
> Estragon: "Yes, let's go" [They do not move]
>
> (Beckett, 1956/2012)

So many of his characters have either ailments or circumstances that keep them trapped in their situations physically or emotionally. In this regard,

Beckett directly challenges the ideals of the self pivoted upon a progressive trajectory of action, productivity, and movement. His characters are generally non-productive in various senses of the word, either through complete stasis in the environment or as paragons of non-reproductivity, where references to love and sex do not conform to narratives of normativity. We can ask why ideals of the body circulate around action and movement in the world in ways that are socially acceptable, such as 'working hard', being athletic, being productive, being reproductive, being helpful to others, and so on. While the concept of autonomy is highly valued, as Goodley argues, it may also be because qualities related to the preferred version of the self contain a notion of movement, dynamism, and directional process: "The processes of biopower have in mind a preferred psychology and version of the self: healthy, rational, autonomous, educated, economically viable, self-governing and able—a self-contained individual" (Goodley, 2011, p. 164)

Of course, we can look at it from an evolutionary perspective, and we might see the body that cannot move as likely to be prey for a hunting animal. Our ability to engage the fight-or-flight mechanism is inherent to our capacity to move freely and react spontaneously to threats. Furthermore, from a biological perspective, we, as human beings, are designed to move our bodies. This makes sense even from a machinic point of view: we need to drive our vehicles to keep them in working order, to keep them from rusting, from failing. When it comes to attitudes towards movement, I think evolutionary perspectives cannot be ignored, despite the gymnastics of discursive perspectives, but they are not an excuse for the narratives that form as a result of the stigma of not doing or doing differently in a conventional sense. We may be primed towards continuous movement and thought in some kind in evolutionary terms or to cover over the pain of existing, but it is important to remember, as Cohen (2019) points out, that we are also driven or impelled toward inactivity, the reduction of tension, the nirvana principle of the zero state of agitation and desire.

Although not necessarily specific to disability, I am building a case for the responses to action and inaction, will and the absence of volition, within the narrative constructions that develop around bodies that are not simply disabled but also different in their manifestation of doing. This will be a useful distinction in considering issues of the body that border on but are not collapsible with disability, but still would be marginalised or alienated through the defiles of ableism, as we will see with the static, hemmed-in bodies in Beckett's work and the inspiration for bodies without organs in Artaud's writings and theatre. In our contemporary times, socially and culturally, doing is clearly valued over being, movement over stasis. Yet, Beckett and Artaud, in different ways through the positioning and representation of the non-normative body, can help us think about being. The typical refrain of contemporary professional subjects, stating how busy they are, feeds into the terrain of attitudes that belie belief in the idealised subject of twenty-first-century capitalism. It is good to be busy, not slothful or wasteful. In contrast to this valorisation of activity and productivity, I think here of the stories of sages who have retired to mountaintops to consider the question of being and the nature of the self, asking the rhetorical and infinite question 'who am I?', and some of whom, according to anecdotal tales, have spent their time watching mindless movies while not doing very much else other than being still. The art of self-reflection requires a certain slowing down, a stopping of frenetic activity in order to cultivate the ability to listen internally to our feelings and thoughts. This slowing down can lead us not to discover who we are in an epiphany of self-realisation, but to a knowledge of the limits of how we know ourselves. In keeping with the philosophy of Geulincx and Rabaté's (2016) exposition of the art of the non relation, we know ourselves through not knowing, through a humility born of an encounter with the limits of existence. While it may seem that the analysis is moving away from an exploration of ableism, we are actually stepping into yet another critique of a tenet of contemporary capitalism's privileging of the autonomous, self-sufficient body: the notion that knowledge is power.

## Narratives of Knowing

The able body is also a body that seemingly has acquired enough knowledge or *savoir faire* to operate self-sufficiently in the world and is a body that has the capacity to increasingly add to the store of knowledge acquisition and production, unlike those who may have succumbed to the pathology of being epistemologically disabled, a theme already mentioned. In other words, in order to arrive at something relatively truthful from a psychoanalytic perspective, we must problematise the question of knowledge and recognise that knowledge is not always power but seduction; its charms can lead us somewhat astray in conceptualising pathways through a dilemma or problematic of experience. We live in a world where science and empirical data are treasured (and with good reason, as without them a certain chaos of speculation would abound) as providing the means of certainty and reassurance to many of life's dilemmas, yet there are domains where this view renders experience which is not empirically verifiable null and of less value. In linking the question of knowledge to the valorisation of the able body, we can outline some of the traits that are deemed, without conscious attribution, to be the cause and sustenance of this autonomous body. A body that functions in a way that produces in a socially normative context is understood to be driven by knowledge and productive of knowledge, and therefore, aspersions are made as to the mind of this person. And by consequence, aspersions are made in a negative light towards the mind of a person deemed to fall from the ideal of knowledge or what we could also call 'body know-how'. As Nobus and Quinn explain:

> The epistemological drive produces an economy in which the formula of 'knowledge is power' is altered; instead, power is used as a means of generating

> knowledge. The mind becomes the metaphorical generator of knowledge in quantity and of quality. It is idealised as productive, and anything that calls a halt to this production is seen as personal tragedy and social waste.
>
> (Nobus and Quinn, 2015, p. 151)

Interestingly, from the perspective of ableism, Nobus and Quinn continue their argument by using the example of the film *A Beautiful Mind* about the economist, mathematician, and game theorist John Nash, who had psychosis, to illustrate their point that interpretations of the film privilege the narrative of a linear progression of health/recovery (in this case, of the mind) toward the value of productivity, knowledge over non-knowledge, or what they call "the 'recovery' of mind and the restoration of value" (2015, p. 152). They argue that the actual reality of John Nash's life was not this straightforward, progressive narrative of recovery of mind and restoration of previous value, but more existed within a partial recovery, where the notion of production through knowledge is problematised. We can see that knowledge is an important factor in identifying the problem with narratives of the body, and that presumptions of knowledge-as-power can underlie narratives of the mind over matter, a perspective so prevalent in twenty-first-century culture.

This discussion of the fall in knowledge, or the failure of the productive narrative of the subject, creates an interesting link with the concept of failure as an epistemological drive in the work of Beckett and Artaud. That is, in some respects, Beckett's work leads us to consider a truth of being as a phenomenon of the body's failing, or, more broadly, as a question of knowledge exposed through a lacking other. If we think of *Waiting for Godot* and the classic question of who Godot really is, despite the fact that Vladimir and Estragon don't know either, we can see quite directly how a question of knowledge is subverted or refracted back at the audience. What *Waiting for Godot* is really about may be a question that arises for people, and the fact that it is about waiting for nothing in particular and, critically, without knowledge of something particular, seems not to satisfy initially until the existential consequence of this theme is fully cognised.

Regarding Artaud's quest for a state of being untainted by the rationalising force of language, while I could be accused of reading an artist's biography too literally as a projection within his writings, I think that Artaud's specific biographical details, his lack of theatrical productions (relatively speaking), and the content of his letters and short prose lends itself to this assumption and to the grapplings with being that his work opens onto. The Theatre of Cruelty appears to capture the imagination in its conceptualisation rather than in its execution, and this is a very curious point. Artaud's theatrical vision, as an experiment in creating a new language of being, in accessing the inaccessible, and in attempting to access the unconscious (through his own conception), is more interesting and provocative in theatre studies than the actuality of the productions. In some respects, this resembles the space of psychoanalysis, where we have most access to the theory of the unconscious rather than its actuality. This also brings us to a problem in applying psychoanalysis to theory or to literature as a means of illuminating or interpreting data in order to arrive at a conclusion or to produce a product of knowledge, a deeper insight into the meaning of literature, albeit provisional. I do not profess to have resolved this contradiction in this book, but the content is certainly informed by this conundrum and the fallout of writing academically through the use of psychoanalysis. And yet, this is where the work of Beckett and Artaud prevents a wholesale application of inert a priori theory and lends itself to what I hope is a more dialectical exploration of the epistemology of the body, where the shadowy borderline between meaning and non-meaning is delineated. Not unlike what Rabaté (2016) calls Beckett's "ethics of the non relation", the ethic underpinning the exploration of the body here is the admission of the power of not knowing and the driving force it creates. In essence, an epistemology of the body in the work of these authors will open interesting avenues for intersectional and dialectical analysis. We will see that what we have discovered about the body in Beckett's and Artaud's dramatic work will form a bridge, elaborating on and adding value to this dialogue on the critique of body–mind narratives, and will serve to challenge some of the simplifications or latent assumptions that influence attitudes across multiple fields. Although writing in a time that preceded the advent of the movement that became disability studies towards the end of the twentieth century, their work is of great interest in this regard, not as I have been arguing as a direct representation of disability, although it can be argued this is a feature of Beckett's work, but as a means of providing tropes, situations that reflect the complexity inherent to the contingent property of embodiment, and, most importantly, the suffering related to these contingencies, a contingency being in my view that of existence itself. Indeed the body itself is, to some degree, not only an ontological feature of embodied being but a contingency of existence in the sense that our embodied states are subject to chance, circumstance, geographical location, and other determinants of our relative positionality in the world. From a psychoanalytic viewpoint, the experience of embodiment is based on an ontological trauma constitutive of existence, rather than a contingent one, though contingent bodily traumas also impact the human subject. While the idea of trauma as a constituent element of our being is not new in psychoanalysis, and certainly not in Lacanian studies, as it occupies a dominant paradigm of subject causation, mapping this critical existential factor of life onto a theorisation of the body while complexifying this relation with the 'mind' brings to the fore theorisations of bodily alterity.

Nonetheless, it is important not to inadvertently idealise the state of the unknown and to acknowledge that if we think of how knowledge is connected within colonial contexts, the body being one of these overlaps, not knowing and the drive to know can create violence, trauma, uncanny effects, hierarchical power dynamics, anxiety, discrimination, and prejudice. While this book does not focus on the elaboration of the implications of the body within colonial or post-colonial contexts, it is certainly worth keeping in mind as one of the ways the human subject responds to the innate trauma of the body. How do we deal with the enigma of our being? The next chapter takes up this question.

## Notes

1 The category of 'disability' is as much a narrative as it is a social construction (Purcell, 2018, p. 16).
2 Freud (1923) "The ego is ultimately derived from bodily sensations, chiefly from those springing from the surface of the body. It may thus be regarded as a mental projection of the surface of the body, besides, as we have seen above, representing the superficies of the mental apparatus."
3 "The Flemish philosopher fully deployed an ethics of humility and impotence, the emergence of which had been prepared by the inversion of Cartesian rationalism into an utter non-knowing. If 'I err, therefore I am', such an erring then generates an ethics of nonvalue" (Rabaté, 2016, p. 68).

## References


Beckett, S. (1958/2012). Endgame. In *Samuel Beckett: The complete dramatic works.* Faber & Faber.

Beckett, S. (1956/2012). Waiting for Godot. In *Samuel Beckett: The complete dramatic works.* Faber & Faber.

Cohen, J. (2019). *Not working: Why we have to stop.* London: Granta Books.

Damasio, A. (1999). *The feeling of what happens: Body and emotion in the making of consciousness.* Mariner Books.

Emanuel, C. (2022). A white and nondisabled psychoanalyst: Owning racism and ableism in the clinical process. *Psychoanalysis, Self and Context*, 17:2, 181–195.

Freud, S. (1923). The Ego and the Id. *The standard edition of the complete psychological works of Sigmund Freud, Volume XIX (1923–1925): The Ego and the Id and Other Works*, 1–66.

Goodley, D. (2011). *Disability studies: An interdisciplinary introduction.* London: Sage Publications.

Harrington, A. (2008). *The cure within: A history of mind–body medicine.* New York & London: Norton.

Harrington, A. (2019). *Mind fixers: Psychiatry's troubled search for the biology of mental illness.* Norton.

Kahneman, D. (2011). *Thinking fast and slow.* New York: Straus and Giroux.

Lacan, J. (2006). *Écrits: The first complete edition in English* (B. Fink, Transl.). New York: W. W. Norton & Company.

Leader, D. (2007). *Why do people get ill? Exploring the mind–body connection.* Hamish Hamilton.

Meehan O'Callaghan, S. (2024). The price of freedom: On not giving ground relative to desire. In C. Owens (Ed.) *Studying Lacan's Seminar VII: The Ethics of Psychoanalysis.* Routledge.

Mollow, A. (2015). *The disability drive*, Unpublished thesis. University of California, Berkeley.
Nobus & Quinn. (2005). *Knowing nothing, staying stupid: Elements of a psychoanalytic epistemology*. Sussex: Routledge.
Purcell, S. (2018). *"Extraordinary debilities": Disability in the works of Samuel Beckett*. Unpublished PhD Thesis NUIG: Galway.
Rabaté, J.M. (2016). *Think, pig! Beckett at the limit of the human*. New York: Fordham University Press.
Shildrick, M. (2009). *Dangerous discourses of disability, subjectivity and sexuality*. London: Palgrave Macmillan.
Verhaeghc, P. (2014). *What about me? The struggle for identity in a market-based society*. (J. Hedley-Prole, Transl.) London: Scribe.

Chapter 3

# The Trauma of the Body

## A Fissure in Being

So far in this book, the body has been framed as a question rather than a definition, reflecting the body's ontological ambiguity in the life of the subject. The last chapter identified some of the ways in which more complex accounts of embodiment that resist binary reductionisms are eschewed in favour of narratives that provide cultural or individual templates of meaning. A semblance of meaning gives us some purchase on the facticity or 'thereness' of our bodies; without it, the body can seem alien, anxiety-provoking, and Other. For example, we often have, consciously or unconsciously, routines and structures within which we operate to contain the body, whether through physical exercise, work, or particular social activities. Although these activities also operate on our psychical and emotional states, they also manage the body as an organism, providing an avenue of release for excitations and drives and a certain palliation of the anxiety of existing through finding meaning in doing. This is why a subject confronted with a rupturing bodily event through accident, illness, or disability can be thrown into disarray or confronted with an alienation of bodily experience. It is not that these situations are the only times when alienation or trauma concerning the body is encountered; we can think of many symptomatic examples within neurotic and psychotic structures, but they are privileged sites for exploring this idea, as often a person's whole world or the meaning structures that support existence are turned upside down. These meaning structures are mediated by fantasies that shield us from the abyss of being, fantasies that surround ideals of a normal body, perpetuated by ableist narratives. This chapter analyses why the body is traumatic and its implications in the field of the arts, employing Lacan's concepts of the object a, fantasy, trauma, and the imaginary. I argue we can read for an aesthetic of the body in both authors' works that, at its heart, concerns a relation to the object a as an analogue of the trauma of the body and the remainder of being.

While the body in Lacan's work is a topic of great enigma and warrants a full exploration across his oeuvre, this book can only point to the complexity of its composition and to its incompleteness as a subject. For example, as psychoanalysts and scholars such as Verhaeghe (2001) and Soler (1984) have

DOI: 10.4324/9781003509622-5

pointed out, there are distinctive shifts in Lacan's conception of the body in the seminars of the 1950s, 60s, and 70s. In the Lacan of the 50s, the imaginary holds sway as giving the body an illusory consistency; in the 60s, the symbolic is more determining (the body is a body of signifiers), and in the Lacan of the 70s, the Real and the jouissance of the body as that which enjoys itself is to the fore.

Therefore, any apparent definitions of concepts have to be considered in the light of the shifting sands of Lacanian chronology. Also, as there is no unified or totalising Lacanian theory (Nobus, 1998, p. xi), we cannot simply apply a ready-made model that would yield a priori knowledge. Although I have not specifically encountered the phrase 'the body is traumatic' in Lacan's work, I wish to argue that this idea is embedded in fundamental concepts of Lacanian theory. As I have already said, Lacan has at times argued that we cannot say exactly what a living body is, and by doing so, he draws into question both the meaning of living substance and the body itself. In *Seminar 21, Les Non Dupes Errent* (1973–1974), Lacan gives one of his most succinct, though still opaque, definitions of the body as an "enjoying substance," something that enjoys itself (Lacan, 13 November 1973, p. 172). While there is a view that the body for Lacan is a construct (Soler, 1984), through which we have a relation of having (Miller, 2010), we can also read it as a phenomenon of being, that which we *are*, albeit as a vacillating concept in his later work.

## A Divide in Being

As I have already outlined, the psychoanalytical human subject is divided, split and decentred in relation to the 'I' of the Cartesian *cogito*. For the Cartesian subject, thought, as that conscious representative of the subject, provides the bedrock or proof of the certainty of existence. Lacan reverses the logic of the Cartesian *cogito ergo sum* and thought becomes the antithesis of being. It is both important and curious to note how prevalent references to Descartes are in Lacan's work, indicating his importance either as a backdrop or a point of departure in theorising what we could call the modern post-structuralist subject. Although Lacan is continuously revising Descartes, he credits him in *Seminar IX, Identification* for bringing the concept of the modern subject into being, though not in the linguistically inflected way that Lacan devises. The fact that the unconscious splits the subject into the ego and the subject of the unconscious has important implications for thinking about the relation between body and mind, and for how we relate to our bodies as both objects of perception and agents of feeling. I have already said that these terms are slippery, and the concept of the subject cannot be anchored in concrete meaning, as it is that which only becomes known through slips in meaning. The Lacanian subject has no essence or substance, nothing that could be classified as material and concrete; it is, in fact, how

Lacan describes the unconscious in *Seminar XI* as pre-ontological, that which has no essence, no inherent substance (1964, p. 29). It is what Verhaghe calls an "indeterminate non-being which can only give rise to an identity, an ego, in retrospect (1998, p. 13).

The fact that the human being is what Lacan (1972–1973) will later refer to as a speaking being implies the critical presence of language within the very 'substance' of our existence. The 'essence' of being is tied to the role of the signifier in cultivating or giving 'birth' to the subject. As Lacan says, "if he did not speak, he would not have the word being" (Lesson VI, 18 February 1975).

That is to say, if we obtain our being from the fact that we speak, the very concept of being is a function of language. The subjection of the human subject to language takes place even before birth through the signifiers significant others use to refer to us. We are in part the effect of the signifier: "It is from the effect of the signifier that the subject as such emerges." (Lacan, Lesson IV, 6 December 1961, p. 30). I say in part, as I do not adhere completely to the idea that our existence is purely a function of signification or, possibly more accurately, 'signifierness' (Lacan, 1972). This will become clearer in later chapters and in Part 3, when I investigate how the body is also a source of being, but for the moment, I want to remain with an earlier Lacanian account of being, that of the being of the subject of the unconscious.

Lacan's definition of a signifier is pretty much a definition of the subject. "A signifier is that which represents a subject for another signifier" (Lacan, 1964, p. 207). The subject exists in the interstices of the signifiers; it has no essential substantive being. In conceptualising being as a function of language and not as pure immanence (a natural substance), Lacan's ideas at this point differ from materialistic conceptions of being, such as within Artaud's aesthetic, where being might be understood to be a direct consequence of the physical body. This is admittedly a somewhat tricky idea, as I have already said; there is no subject without a body, and yet, as I understand it from Lacan's language-oriented perspective on the unconscious, we, our being as subjects, are not completely reduced to it.

The Lacanian subject of the unconscious challenges the fantasy and cultural ideal of an autonomous, self-governing subject who masters the vicissitudes of the body by strengthening the ego. While other therapies (including post-Freudian ego psychology) aimed at reinforcing the ego through identification with the therapist, underlying a belief in the rational and conscious self, where the I of the statement is taken to refer to a knowable entity, Lacan categorically rejected the notion of object relations, or a state where we 'overcome' our problems through reality adaptation. It is not through identification that we obtain freedom but through a beyond of identification, one which can leave us confronted with great anguish. in *Seminar VII, The Ethics of Psychoanalysis*, he emphasises a tragic dimension to the process of analysis, where the subject encounters a disarray through analysis—what has become referred to at the end of analysis as "subjective destitution" (Verhaeghe and Declercq, 2002, p. 11). While psychoanalysis aims to disentangle the subject from the desire of the Other (through the process of speaking and scanning the unconscious) and to allow for a subjectivation of desire as singular, this is not a freedom based on finding the last word on oneself or on finding a meaning to life. On the contrary, as Beckett encountered through texts such as *The Unnamable,* there can be no 'last word' to the articulations of the subject, no point at which the question of 'who am I' is answered adequately. The ground is always shifting beneath the personal pronoun. The very structure of the signifier, as it continuously slips between meanings, between other signifiers, proves that the 'last word' on any subject is impossible. It is also what prevents us from having a unified concept of body and mind; instead, we must deal with a more fragmented and complex entity, often oversimplified through narratives of wholeness or fragmentation. The body is not whole but is a body with 'holes' or, as Brenner puts it in his discussion of the autistic body 'without holes,' erotogenic organs (2021, p.48). These holes relate to the Real of the body not being fully assimilated by the symbolic and presuppose a traumatic residue at the level of bodily substance.

This idea of trauma as endogenous differs from traditional and chronologically inflected notions of trauma as a trace or rupture in the present that marks the impact of a past event. It originally stems from Freud's theory of the drive/drives, where the drives, as internal sources of tension, can overwhelm the subject and be experienced as traumatic—trauma being that excess of excitation which breaches the ego defences either externally or internally. Interestingly, in *Project for a Scientific Psychology* (1895) and in *Beyond the Pleasure Principle* (1920), Freud refers to trauma as pain, which forges an important connection between states of illness, pain, disability, and trauma.[1] In Lacanian terms, the drives, although related to the signifier, are pathways to the Real of the body: they are sources of jouissance that, through a Freudian lens, can have a traumatic dimension. In *The Four Fundamental Concepts of Psychoanalysis,* the Real is already clearly linked to trauma:

> What is repeated, in fact, is always something that occurs [...] as if by chance. [...] The function of the tuché, of the real as encounter—the encounter in so far as it may be missed, in so far as it is essentially the missed encounter—first presented itself in the history of psycho-analysis in a form that was in itself already enough to arouse our attention, that of the trauma. Is it not remarkable that, at the origin of the analytic experience, the real should have presented itself in the form of that which is unassimilable in it—in the form of the trauma, determining all that follows, and imposing on it an apparently accidental origin?
>
> (Lacan, 1964, pp. 54-55)

Lacan is here drawing on the Aristotelian concepts of automaton and tuche, where automaton relates to the network of signifiers that encircles the void of meaning and tuche the Real. A connection is forged between chance, the Real, and trauma; the Real presents itself 'in the form of' a trauma. From this perspective, an encounter with the Real is a missed encounter, something that by its very nature does not add up. As the Real is that aspect of human experience which resists symbolisation or is in excess of language, the nature of this missed encounter cannot be represented in words. Rather it ex-ists as the impossible dimension of the subject. As a function of the missed encounter, the Real is "that which always comes back to the same place—the place where the subject does not meet it" (Lacan, 1964/1978, p. 49). Fundamentally, the missed encounter is that of the signifier and the Real, and this missed encounter occurs 'as if by' chance.[2] In other words, it is not a chance encounter, but it often appears to be this way. Think of the accidental character of a parapraxis, a slip of the tongue, a forgetting of a name. Critically, Lacan's account of the Real as trauma is a trauma that differs from a narrative of a traumatic event. As Gil Caroz explains, "[Lacan] somehow purifies the Freudian theory of trauma. He empties it of the drama and the story that surrounds it and makes of the trauma a moment of encounter between the body and a trace of the signifier" (Caroz, n. d, p. 4). In other words, the missed encounter is the impossibility of the human subject to ever encounter the cause of being, as the cause is paradoxically both structural and yet outside the subject. This impossibility is identifiable through the act of repetition. As Lacan argues, trauma is marked by the mechanism of repetition compulsion, but repetition can only repeat something as a missed encounter; it can never actually be or fully represent the traumatic event itself. There is always a remainder in repetition, something that cannot be repeated but that drives the impetus to repeat. I will return to the idea of repetition in the next chapter, considering the repeated presence of truncated or fragmented bodies in Beckett's oeuvre and how this serves as a stylistic leitmotif that reveals a fantasy about the body. Ironically, this is not a fantasy of the body as 'normal' but as debilitated—a pathway to access the truth of being. This truth, however, due to the presence of the unconscious, is based on a discord of being, something that doesn't add up or is impossible to access.

## The Unconscious and the Body: A Fundamental Discord

We recall that incorporating the unconscious into the question of the body enables us to move beyond the binary of the mind–body paradigm and adopt a more complex account of subjectivity, where multiple elements are at play beyond the simple dichotomy of two separate, reciprocal, or non-reciprocal substances. However, it is not clear how the unconscious relates to a body, or what implications this has for lived reality.

As a concept (and indeed as a phenomenon), the unconscious is not easy to 'locate' theoretically or topographically (particularly as something of the unconscious lies outside representation) but Lacan has at times given clear definitions of the unconscious. Fundamentally, and somewhat counter-intuitively, the unconscious is something that is outside the subject: "The unconscious is the discourse of the Other … Now, the discourse of the Other that is to be realized, that of the unconscious, is not beyond the closure, it is *outside* " (1964, p. 134). Thus, rather than existing in a locatable psychic space, the unconscious manifests as a phenomenon of discontinuity within lived experience: "Discontinuity then, is the essential form in which the unconscious first appears to us as a phenomenon—discontinuity, in which something is manifested as a vacillation" (ibid, p. 25). Lacan explains that the unconscious is not something clear-cut, but rather functions as that cut, a discontinuity within the conventions of meaning, resulting in a rupture or vacillation of sense or what, in Freudian terms, is called a parapraxis. In this way, the unconscious operates as a "rupture, split" (ibid, p. 26); it is in the flash of this momentary opening and closing that the subject of the unconscious reveals itself. Lacan's conception of the unconscious differed from Freud's, most notably in the nature of its structure. For Lacan, the unconscious is not a basement space full of repressed desires but instead exists as a curve in space and time, functioning within language as an Other space.[3]

As this Other space, the unconscious as a discontinuity, a "gap", an "unpublished word" (Lacan, Lesson 10, 16 June 1971), marks the divide of the subject (of the unconscious) from the body. The relationship of the unconscious to the body is one of discontinuity, and this discontinuity will always subvert a stable or reliable conception of what a body is within the realm of meaning. As Lacan says:

> There is nothing in the unconscious—if it is made as I have stated to you—that makes an agreement with the body. The unconscious is discordant. The unconscious is that which, by speaking, determines the subject as being, but being to be removed from this metonymy, by which *I* support desire, as forever impossible to say as such.
>
> (Lacan, Lesson 4, 22 January 1974–75)

So the subject is determined as a being but a being whose body does not align with it in any speakable way, it would seem. This is surely problematic at the level of lived existence, as it indicates a certain emptiness at the heart of a living substance. It also doesn't define what a body is. As Rik Loose argues (2002):

> Language, therefore, constitutes a subject and a body, but not in the same place—the subject is not the body. Where the subject is, we find no-body; and where the body is, we find no subject. Despite this fundamental disjunction there is a relationship but it is problematic in nature.
>
> (p. 179)

We can hear the diminutive evocations of nobody in the subject's place; the subject is not a someone, a specific so-and-so, but a nobody, a void, a substanceless signifier. According to Loose, a sobering consequence of the division of the body into the Real and the symbolic is that the subject literally feels torn apart, rendered somewhat asunder by the signifier, which is the "destiny of the human subject" (2002, p. 188).

The implications of the disjunction between subject and body raise many questions about the being of the subject and that of the body. From what Lacan says here, the subject of the unconscious seems almost disembodied; yet surely this is impossible, as the body or at least the organism gives birth to the subject. Several questions arise: does the unconscious have a physical/organic correlate or is it somehow outside physicality? Is the subject of the unconscious also a subject of the body, or is it purely of the signifier, given its initial sparking through the life-giving force of the body? And by body, do we mean the organism or the symbolic and imaginary body, in part a linguistic construct? It is not easy to answer this definitively, but perhaps the subject is divided relative to the unconscious and the body: there is a subject of the body and a subject of language, or what I would call a being of the body and a being of the subject. Language may establish a body but it cannot completely pacify it. I will return to this idea later in the book but it is important to establish that body and mind do not add up to a unity—ultimately, If the subject and the body are not constituted in the same place, or even if the subject of the unconscious has no body, there can never be a direct synchrony of 'body and mind', layers of identification (related to the ego, the imaginary order and the symbolic; ideal ego and ego-ideal), cover or veil the discord between subject and body. These binary terms are inherently problematic, as, according to Lacan's terminology, the unconscious cannot be reduced to the mind in an individual sense, as it ex-ists 'outside'.

In essence, then, at the level of the signifier or the signifying chain, there is something that appears to live on independently of the body. As something of the subject is borne of the signifying chain, then the subject does not die completely with the death of the body; at the very least, traces of it remain with the symbolic (Soler, 1984). We must stop here again to reconsider the question of the body; what body are we referring to? Is it one of flesh and blood, that which we feel as pain, enjoyment, or pleasure, that which we see in the mirror or that which we refer to in language? I think that the body is a function of the three registers: the imaginary, the real, and the symbolic, and therefore we can deduce that it exists on all these levels, which makes it hard to refer to as one signifier. However, the later Lacan places the consistency of the body more in the imaginary (Collins, 2024) than in the symbolic, a shift from the earlier theory of the mirror phase, in which the body is more an imagistic form than anything substantive. Although we need to remember what I previously quoted, Lacan says we don't know what a living body is, but that it is something that enjoys itself. This enjoyment is, as I understand it, the Real of the organism at the level of jouissance. Colette Soler makes the point that the body is not just a product of the imaginary but also is a "drive-ridden body" (Soler, 2016, p. 52). Of course, perhaps it is a question of how we conceive of the imaginary that is at stake in conceptualising the body as an identification at the level of having, or as a substance at the level of being.

We will continuously come back to the prevalence of the imaginary in conceptualising a body, but for the moment, let us consider the implications for how, at its core, if we can say such a thing, given something of the core may be outside, there is a traumatic kernel of the Real. While the symbolic provides an organisation of this Real through the cuts of signifiers that form a body, the imaginary order protects us from the '*horror vacui*' of this ontological void, providing a sense of grounding and anchoring in meaning through identifications that are rooted both in the Real of the body and the imagistic register. In *Seminar XXII, RSI,* Lacan refers to the imaginary as that which gives consistency and substance—something that is different from the earlier illusory context of the imaginary. "There is no Imaginary which does not suppose a substance" (Lacan, Lesson 2, 17 December 1974–1975). While the idea of substance is a later conception of the imaginary, returning to the imaginary's earlier status in Lacan's theory of the mirror stage is also helpful for tracing the different dimensions of identification or Otherness concerning the body in Lacan's theory and its wide-ranging applications. Certainly theories of the mirror stage still abound as proffered explanations for why the body in states of alterity can pose such discord—the non-normative body defies the so-called Gestalt in the mirror—but these theories tend not to rely on conceptions of identification as visual/ specular when in fact identification and feelings of discord have much deeper roots.

## The Imaginary and its Deformations

As the mirror stage is well known, I will not go into too much detail here but will contextualise its relevance to conceptions of the body and its implications within the field of the arts and spectatorship. In essence, the mirror stage accounts for the structural alienation of the human subject within the symbolic order, an alienation that is predicated on an introjected image of a false self. The mirror stage refers to a period in a young child's life when they look in the mirror or at another person and recognise themselves as the reflection of their own body. The mirror image provides the preliminary physical correlate of the one who says 'I'—a seeming appearance of a substance. This pivotal misrecognition is the seat from which binary assumptions about self and other, and subsequent identifications, are made.

In *The Mirror Stage as Formative of the I Function* (1949), Lacan outlines the relationship between the child's body and the specular image reflected in the mirror. This image is assumed to be the subject, yet it is only a reflection. As he says:

> The jubilant assumption[assumption] of his specular image by the kind of being—still trapped in his motor impotence and nursing dependence—[...] by which he must resolve, as I, his discordance with his own reality.
>
> (1949/2004, p. 4)

As this suggests, the mirror stage marks a fundamental discord between the interior self and the specular image. The specular image serves as a Gestalt (unified image) with which the child begins to identify. This specular Gestalt is the introjection of an image that appears as a whole entity and paradoxically creates both unity and chaos. The term Gestalt derives from a German word meaning form. Thus in the dialectic of the mirror stage, the outer form of the body is interpreted as an organised entity, serving to placate the inner helplessness of the formless interior. The discord concomitant with this process is referred to as a *meconnaisance*, or misrecognition, between the ego and the image, a misrecognition that leads to varying conflicts concerning aggression and rivalry. The 'I' is taken to be the 'me' that is reflected in the mirror and all future I statements are predicated on this seminal identification. The 'I' is an Other as Rimbaud said. This point of discordant identification is the seat of all future identifications; there will always be a gap between the ideal ego (narcissistic image) and the ego-ideal (external world). The ideal ego refers to the primary narcissistic identification with a self-image that forms the basis of all future identifications, whereas the ego-ideal is the introjection of an image or a signifier from the symbolic order and a primary significant other. According to Chiesa:

> the ego-ideal is the subject's introjection of another external image that has a new (de)formative effect on his psyche. In other words, the ego-ideal adds to the ego a new stratum that provides the subject with a secondary identification.
>
> (Chiesa, 2007, p 22)

Chiesa makes a critical point here about how, paradoxically, the imaginary can affect change in the imaginary dimension of subjectivity, and I will return to this when discussing how art/theatre can shape or change us through deformations of the imaginary.

While all these concepts require more rigorous examination than can be provided here, a key point to bear in mind is the implications for the question of the body.

For the Lacan of the 1940s, the material body (as image) is complicit in the alienating constitution of ego identity; it is part of the exterior illusion that becomes introjected as a seemingly stable image of what the 'moi' or self is. As Lacan says:

> For the total form of his body, by which the subject anticipates the maturation of his power in a mirage, is given to him only as a gestalt,

> that is in an exteriority in which, to be sure, this form is more constitutive than constituted.
>
> (Lacan, 1949/2004, p. 4)

The form, or the image of the body, allows the subject to relate to the body as if it were a solid entity, constituting an unstable sign of who I am. Yet this stability or Gestalt takes place at the level of the ego, not at the level of the subject, if we apply the idea that the subject and the body are not in the same place. In this way, the body and the ego are intimately connected within the dialectic of misrecognition—where 'I' is another body. This seems to explain why there can be such narcissistic devastation when changes to the appearance of the body or to the body's functioning occur—as the theory goes, the imaginary Gestalt is no longer working to shield the subject from the internal chaos of the drives. However, these theories rely too much on Lacan's early thinking on the imaginary and not enough on the introduction of the object a as that distortion in the field of the visible. I think we can take this further to consider how sensations of the body, pain, jouissance, and affect also dysregulate the subject at the level of being without necessarily a visible, specular dimension at play. In other words, who we are is also related to a felt sense, an affectual dimension, something that has no specular image but causes a distortion or discordance with what we can say or see of ourselves.

While the mirror stage depicts a scenario of seduction with an image of who we are, it has also been a seductive theory within the arts for explaining the dynamics of identification a little too neatly. As Todd McGowan explains (2007) in *The Real Gaze,* early Lacanian theory in film studies focused largely on how the mirror stage provided a means to explain how subjects were interpellated by ideology through vectors of identification and created an alignment of cinema as an imaginary pleasure. However, these early theorists were limited in situating the gaze purely in the realm of the spectator and did not take into account Lacan's later theory of the gaze as an object in the real. For McGowan, the gaze as object a paves the way to disentangle some of the problematics associated with the look of the spectator and assess the particularities of a film: "It is not the look of the subject at the object, but the gap within the subject's seemingly omnipotent look" (2007, p. 6).

The introduction of the gaze shifts the theory of the imaginary away from the human subject's identification with the image, to a subversion of identification within the image (caused by a lack within the specular). Hence, the application of the gaze in the field of the arts allows for a subversion of binary formulations of spectatorship, in which the look is deemed to be on the side of the spectator and egoic identification is a potential consequence of the artistic encounter. Lacan, on the other hand, positions the gaze in the field of the Other. In contrast to the concept of the gaze in Sartre, it is "not a seen gaze, but a gaze imagined by me in the field of the Other" (Lacan, 1964, p. 84). The gaze "is that underside of consciousness" (ibid, p. 83), which is outside the visual object but inside, as something that lures us to look. The gaze is the object a in the field of the visible, a lack induced by the split of the divided subject, where desire circulates around a nothingness framed by an image: "The objet a in the field of the visible is the gaze" (ibid, p. 105).

While I find Lacan's deployment of the gaze intriguing within the context of the arts, as a point of rupture within the visual image that relates to the body, it also has its limitations and can corral thinking to a particular timeframe of his work.

As Maria Scott (2015) points out, several variations or shifts in Lacan's thinking on the gaze demand closer scrutiny in *Seminar XI, The Four Fundamental Concepts of Psychoanalysis.* While the gaze appears to be on the side of the real as that lost object that cannot be specularised or recovered, it also veers into the imaginary as that object that substitutes for lack. In other words, although apparently an absence, a distortion in the field of the visible, it is something that comes close to being a visible point within the specular field. According to Scott, these variations have led to a lot of confusion regarding their application in film theory. It is important to recognise these vacillations in Lacan's concepts and resist presenting ideas as if they were completely coherent. This involves a certain resistance to the lure of the imaginary as it concerns knowledge, in which theoretical propositions may act as ideational gestalts, causing a certain inertia in thinking and creativity.

Furthermore, although the gaze is one of the avatars of the object a, I do not situate all employments of the object a in this book within the field of the gaze. Despite the emphasis here on spectatorship and the visual/perceptual field, the object a, as it concerns the body, has broader implications within the context of each individual dramatic work. I conceptualise the object a in theatre not simply as a lost object or remainder that sparks the desire of the spectator, so as not solely that of the gaze, but also as a concept that orientates the body within the work of Beckett and Artaud as a question of being—it is their relation to the object a within fantasy that manifests through the decompositions, effacements and idealisations of the body found in their work. In other words, we can elucidate how the body functions as a trauma in their drama by identifying a particular positionality towards the Other, a positionality we need to consider as the relation of the object a within unconscious fantasy.

## Traces of a Body

If body and mind are discordant entities, the object a is a means of speaking about the body as an entity that is not whole but nonetheless leaves a trace, a remainder that is linked to a series of part objects, as in the voice, the gaze, the breast, the phallus. These drive components are both potential triggers of desire and signify the traumatic dimension of the drive, in its potential to overwhelm the subject from within. Speaking very generally, unconscious fantasy is that which orientates the subject of desire vis-à-vis the object a and is a means of protecting ourselves from the trauma of the drive, or in other words, from the real of the body. Fantasy is a subjective construct that positions each subject within the symbolic order as a desiring subject and, as I would see it, is composed of an intersection of the imaginary and the Real at the level of the unconscious. As Chiesa puts it:

> Fantasy has two basic interconnected functions: it both relates the barred subject to the real lack in the Symbolic, that of the real objet a, and, at the same time, 'veils' this lack in the unconscious through the imaginary dimension of the object a.
>
> (2007, p. 142)

In this sense, reality as we know it is refracted mainly through subjective fantasy; hence, reality is a fiction. As we have seen, the experience of embodiment contains a traumatic kernel, as that which signifies a lack of knowledge concerning the body. Fantasy is a veil that covers this hole in knowledge and in this way, it is linked to the imagination as a lining of representation, but is not something that can be directly accessed through words. Lacan's matheme of fantasy is represented by the following:

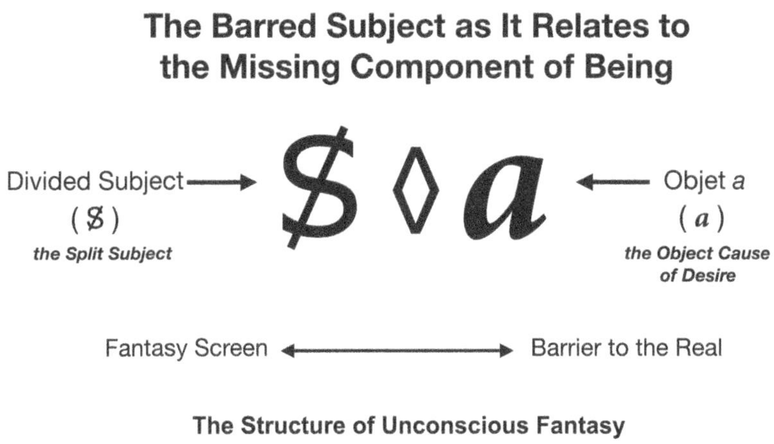


*Figure 3.1* The Structure of Unconscious Fantasy

## The Matheme of Fantasy

The subject is divided in respect of the split of the signifier and fantasy is that which mediates the subject's relationship with the lost object of desire, the object a. Thus, fantasy constructs an orientation of the subject's position in relation to this lost object. In this sense, we could say that through fantasy, we can construct narratives surrounding something that is no longer present but that we wish to experience again. It enables us to touch the impossible, that which is out of reach temporarily and permanently.

It is when fantasy collapses or fails to function that we are exposed to the fissure of being as subjects of language. The object a is not simply representative of a lack at the level of the body, but, if we read it as Lacan describes it at different stages, it signifies an absence at the level of being. The 'a' of object a derives from the French word for other (*autre*), and therefore the loss is related to something that has been subtracted from the field of the Other. As Lacan puts it: "The a is called a in our discourse [...] Because it's what on n'a plus, what we ain't got no more" (Lacan, 1962–1963/2014, p. 117). This missing element or loss is what Lacan refers to as a pound of flesh: "In the body there is always, by virtue of this engagement in the signifying dialectic, something that is separated off, something that is sacrificed, something inert, and this something is the pound of flesh" (ibid, p. 219). As we have seen, the subject is divided through the defiles of the signifier, which separates the conceptual categories of being and existence—a certain amount of being is lost to those who speak (*manque à être*)—as a result of the constitutive cut of language that forms the divided subject. Hence, for the Lacanian subject, existence does not precede essence; there is no essence to being: it is a being which lacks. It is the signifier which precedes existence. So that we can exist within the symbolic and communicate with others, we forego a pound of flesh in the Real. As speaking subjects, therefore, we 'exist' through the signifier while a certain portion of being remains unnameable, unrepresentable and inaccessible to us.

Most importantly for my analysis, the object a is also that which links the body to being: it is "being in so far as it is essentially missing in the text of the world" (Lacan, Lesson XXVI, 22 February 1961–62, p. 308). This is a critical point as it aligns the object a as a signifier of the Real of the body, as that which marks the trauma of the body. As Vanheule (2011) puts it: "The object a refers to the element of the living being that cannot be inserted into the order of the symbolic; a component of flesh and blood that remains inert in relation to the signifier." (p. 131).

By 'locating' this object as irretrievable, never to be refound and forever lost, Lacan conceptualises a structural dissatisfaction inherent to subjectivity and addresses the shortfalls of object relations and phenomenological analyses. This object is not an object that, if found, could satisfy a need, but is instead a remainder, a placeholder marking a cut, a mark on the body of the subject resulting from the encounter with the symbolic order. In this sense, the object a is also defined as the object cause of desire as it drives the metonymical quest from one object to another. This remainder "is what survives the ordeal of the division of the field of the Other through the presence of the subject" (Lacan, 1964/2014, p. 220). In this sense, it cannot be uncovered empirically as if it were an object of specific knowledge. Lacan is explicit:

> This object of desire oughtn't to be confused with the object defined by epistemology. The advent of the object of our science is very specifically defined by a particular discovery of the efficacy of the signifying operation as such.
>
> (ibid, p. 37)

In the realm of sexuality, the object a serves to mark the trauma of the non-rapport of the sexual relationship, where there is always something missing in the so-called idealised sexual union. The non-rapport of the sexual relation subverts traditional ideas of Oneness and complementarity in the vicissitudes of sexual attraction. Rather than supplementing each other in romantic relationships as in one part of a missing half, we are seduced by a quality of lack in the other; something of the Real is touched, that which cannot be captured tangibly. This is how the object cause of desire functions, through enigma, the desire of the Other, but as points of tangency with the body: the gaze, the voice, the mouth, aspects of the body that relate or potentially connect with another.

In the area of sexuality, Lacan opposed conventional psychoanalytic ideas concerning the putative normative trajectory of the sexual drive. Traditional psychoanalytic ideas underscored the view that satisfaction and general happiness in life occurred through a sexual relationship with somebody of the opposite sex. The introduction of the object a as the object of fantasy disturbs this view; total satisfaction is not to be found in the arms of another, as obtaining full satisfaction is impossible due to the primordial loss. There will always be a residue, something that does not add up, something that keeps the human being circling a cause, a traumatic cause of non-meaning.

This concept of that which is 'found' in the object but cannot be seen, the invisible trace of something lost, irretrievable, and yet compelling with regard to knowledge, is crucial to the paradoxes inherent to tracing the trauma of the body in Beckett and Artaud's dramatic works. As we saw earlier, theatre is renowned for certain expressive and phenomenological qualities: the immediacy of performance, presence, liveness, actuality, and embodiment. However, behind the 'reality' of presence lies an equally significant domain of absence, veiled by the plausibility of immediacy. From the spectator's perspective, the body-as-perceived, framed by the fictional dimension of the stage and the aestheticisation of its form, lacks something; a distance is created by the fictional representation. However, this is not a conscious perception of lack, but it enables the enjoyment of the specular image. The object a is something that cannot be represented by an actual body; it is that very part of ourselves that distorts the visible field and prevents us from seeing accurately (McGowan, 2007). In this sense, the body on stage signifies absence as presence through the impossibility of revealing the entirety of experience. As Lacan puts it: "Because of the fact that where he is represented he is absent, that nevertheless being represented, he thus finds himself divided (Lacan, Lesson 1, 1 January 1971). Representation on the stage is therefore paradoxical; wherever the body is present, the subject of the unconscious is also absent or present through a vacillation, a distortion in sense.

Fundamentally, the discord between the unconscious and the body implies that there is no final referent, signified, or meaning that can be attributed to the subject's relationship to the materiality of the flesh, as this discontinuity is inherent to the signifier and the symbolic order within which we are situated in language. The very words we use to describe this materiality bring us both closer to and further away from the Real of the body, or perhaps more accurately, the Real of the flesh. The gap between the materiality of the body as that which is lived (being) and the experience of it as image or signification (as that which we have) is alienating in that, as subjects of language, we are foreclosed from ever joining up with our bodies fully coherently: the body, like the ego, is always, to a degree, Other to us. We are alienated within language but also as subjects with a body.

## Alienation: The I Is an Other (Body)

We are never simply at one with our bodies; there is an inherent estrangement, at times more acute than others. This can be understood in part through the alienation of the subject within language as that which creates a discord with the body. As Martin Jay (2018) has pointed out, Lacan's account of alienation, encapsulated within the poststructuralist turn, differs from that of his philosophical contemporaries and predecessors in envisaging alienation not as pathological and something to be overcome, but as structural and inevitable. In this sense, alienation marks the resistance to conceptions of the self that presume a wholeness or unity is possible or that place alienation in socio-economic terms. In Lacanian terms, alienation is a function of the meaning systems we are born into, both as a consequence of the signifier and the function of the image as a template for the bodily ego. Fundamentally, for Lacan in 1964, alienation represents the 'choice' for a divided subject who is subject to the signifier, caught between meaning and being and between subject and body. Lacan refers to this as the *vel* (Latin word meaning or) of alienation—a forced choice between being and meaning: a choice which is, "neither one, nor the other" (Lacan 1964/1978, p. 211).

If we choose being, we give up the shelter of meaning; if we choose meaning we forgo an aspect of ourselves to the signifiers of the Other—we become mortified by the symbolic. Language is an Other: we have not created the words we use for ourselves; we are born into them, they shape and mould us, causing a split between what is conscious and what is unconscious. This split constitutes an inherent discord, a non-totalising dimension to the 'being of the subject' and the impossibility of ever becoming One.

Essentially, human beings are composed of elements that are both intrinsic and foreign/Other to them. One of these elements of Otherness concerns the body (Canellopoulos, 2010; Verhaeghe, 2001). I take this Otherness to exist at all levels: the Real, as in the organism and jouissance; the imaginary, as in the body image; and the symbolic, as it concerns the signifier. Of course, this may oversimplify things, since the registers overlap and are not strictly separate. It seems that when the body is mentioned even in psychoanalysis, it is hard to specify which body or rather which register of the body, we are referring to. This is partly an issue of the inspecificities of language. For once, we start using signifiers to represent ourselves to others, there will always be something that words or signifiers cannot show; language or images can never fully account for who we are. We are alienated within the very mechanisms of meaning itself, caught within an estrangement of self-knowledge that will remain the basis for further knowledge acquisition (Venheule, 2011, p. 6). In other words, there is always a position of discordance within our relationship to knowledge, and thus the potential to become identified with the products of knowledge; yet this identification can only ever be a *meconnaisance*. While alienation is not specifically traumatic, it can be seen as a response to the trauma of the undifferentiated Real that threatens to engulf a subject. It is perhaps reactionary to an even more primordial split at the level of the living being, a level that Lacan says distinguishes us as sexed beings:

> This lack takes up the other lack, which is the real, earlier lack, to be situated at the advent of the living being, that is to say, at sexed reproduction. The real lack is what the living being loses, that part of himself qua living being, in reproducing himself through the way of sex. This lack is real because it relates to something real, namely, that the living being, by being subject to sex, has fallen under the blow of individual death.
>
> (Lacan, 1964, p. 205)

Thus, the very inception of the living being as a sexed being renders the human subject a being unto death. This real lack is not something produced by language; it precedes it. Language generates another layer of lack, this time within the symbolic, around a cause that cannot be symbolised as it was outside language to begin with. This cause is traumatic: "The introduction of sexuality is traumatizing [...] The central bad encounter is at the level of the sexual" (ibid, p. 64). Sexuality can thus manifest as a trauma of the body, when jouissance as an excess in the body invades the subject and language fails to contain the Real of the non-rapport.

As we can see, trying to establish the body's relation to the unconscious does not lead to easy answers but exposes the complexity and limitations of preexisting theories of embodiment, which fail to account for the Real that cannot be contained within language or a visual image of the body. The trauma of the body captures the varying dimensions of the non-rapport and non-complementarity of the subject's relation to the body across the three registers: the Real, the imaginary, and the symbolic. There is a discord between the subject and the body at the level of the unconscious, the missed encounter between the signifier and the real, the alienation of the ego and the body image, and the non-reciprocity of the sexual relation, which presupposes there is a jouissance at the level of the body that we must endure without satisfaction. Trauma is an ontological phenomenon yet appears through contingencies of chance, and is intrinsic to our very being as subjects of the unconscious. In identifying concepts such as the imaginary, alienation, the object a, the Other, and fantasy as that which implicates the body within the paradigm of the unconscious, we can trace how the body functions within the works of the authors as something both within and beyond its physical form, foregrounding core questions concerning being, a being which does not fit neatly into simplifications of mind–body binaries.

## Notes

1 It is interesting that in *The Book of Love and Pain* (2004), Juan David Nasio points out that there is a lack of devoted study to the subject of pain in psychoanalytic literature. I would ask whether this is related to the intrinsic problems of theorising pain as being outside language. For Nasio, pain has a paradoxical status. It is a limit point, a defence against jouissance, a barrier to an invasion of the drives of the body.

2 It is beyond the scope of this book to extrapolate on the very interesting implications of the intersections of chance, the Real, and the trauma of the body. In Catherine Malabou's book *The New Wounded* (2012), she expands on what she feels to be a neglected component of psychoanalysis, the accidental as trauma within physical states of damage such as Alzheimer's disease.

3 Although still a space of discontinuity, the Freudian unconscious was more topographical than topological. That is to say, it was schematised as more linear and stratified than a space whose shape is continuous and intersecting. In *The Psychopathology of Everyday Life* (1901), Freud analyses the ways in which the unconscious manifests in everyday life. He coined the term parapraxis to designate a phenomenon where the unconscious is manifest as an error in the intended aim, such as a bungled action, a slip of the tongue, or a case of forgetting. A parapraxis denotes where a conscious intention is interrupted by a discontinuity, a presence of something unexpected that throws meaning into question.

## References


Brenner, L. (2021). Is the autistic body a body without organs? In B. McLaughlin & E. Daffron (Eds.) *The body in theory: Essays after Lacan and Foucault*. pp. 42–56. McFarland & Company.

Canellopoulos, L. (2010). The bodily event, jouissance and the (post)modern subject. *Recherches en Psychanalyse, 10 (2)*, 321a–328a. doi:10.3917/rep.010.0141.

Caroz, G. (n.d.). Body event in psychoanalysis. *Irish Circle of Lacanian Orientation*: Retrieved 21 November 2019 from http://iclo-nls.org/?page_id=235.

Chiesa, L. (2007). *Subjectivity and otherness*. New York: The MIT Press.

Collins, D. (2024). Introduction: Debunking the drive. In *Critical essays on the drive: Lacanian theory and practice* (Eds. D. Collins & E. Watson). Routledge.

Freud, S. (1895/1950/2001). Project for a Scientific Psychology. In J. Strachey (Ed.), *The standard edition of the complete psychological works of Sigmund Freud (Vol. 1)* 238–397. London: Vintage.

Freud, S. (1920). *Beyond the pleasure principle*. (Authorised Translation from the 2nd German edition by C.J.M. Hubback). (E. Jones, Ed.) Rosings Digital Publications.

Jay, M. (2018). A history of alienation. *Aeon*. 14 March. Retrieved 1 September 2019 from https://aeon.co/essays/in-the-19505-everybody-cool-was-a-little-alienated-what-changed.

Lacan, J. (1949/2004). The mirror stage as formative of the I function. In B.A. Fink (Ed.), *Ecrits* (pp. 3–9). New York: Norton.

Lacan, J. (1961–1962). *The seminar of Jacques Lacan. Book IX. Identification*. Transl. C. Gallagher. Unpublished.

Lacan, J. (1962–1963/2014). *Anxiety: The seminar of Jacques Lacan, book X*. (J. A. Miller, Ed., & A. Price, Transl.) Cambridge: Polity Press.

Lacan, J. (1964/1978). *The seminar of Jacques Lacan, book XI. The Four Fundamental Concepts of Psychoanalysis*. (J. A. Miller, Ed., & A. Sheridan, Transl.) New York: Norton.

Lacan, J. (1970–1971). *The seminar of Jacques Lacan, book XVIII. On a discourse that might not be a semblance*. (C. Gallagher, Transl.). Unpublished.

Lacan, J. (1972–1973/1999). *Encore. Book XX. On feminine sexuality and the limits of love and knowledge*. (J.-A. Miller, Ed., & B. Fink, Transl.) New York: Norton.

Lacan, J. (1973–1974). *The seminar of Jacques Lacan, book XXI. Les non dupes errent*. (C. Gallagher, Transl.). Unpublished.

Lacan, J. (1974–1975). *The seminar of Jacques Lacan, book XXII. RSI*. Transl. C. Gallagher. Unpublished.

Loose, R. (2002). *The subject of addiction: Psychoanalysis and the administration of enjoyment*. Karnac.

McGowan, T. (2007). *The real gaze*. State University of New York Press.

Miller, J.-A. (1999/2010). Lacanian biology and the event of the body (B. P. Fulks & J. Jauregui, Transl.). *Lacanian Ink*, 18, 7–29.

Nobus, D. (1998). Preface. In D. Nobus (Ed.), *Key concepts of Lacanian psychoanalysis*. New York: Other Press.

Scott, M. (2015). Deciphering the gaze in Lacan's 'of the gaze as objet petit a'. Retrieved 29 November 2019 from http://thedsproject.com/portfolio/decipheting-the-gaze-in-lacans-of-the-gaze-as-objet-petit-a/.

Soler, C. (2016). *Lacanian affects: The function of affect in Lacan's work*. Routledge.

Vanheule, S. (2011). *The subject of psychosis. A Lacanian perspective.* London: Palgrave Macmillan.

Verhaeghe, P. (2019). *Lacan's answer to alienation: Separation.* 365–388. Retrieved 16 November from https://crisisctitique.org/april2019/paul.pdf.

Verhaeghe, P. (1998). Causation and destitution of a pre-ontological non-entity: On the Lacanian subject. In: *Key concepts of Lacanian psychoanalysis*, London: Rebus Press, pp. 164–189. New York: State University of New York Press.

Verhaeghe, P & Declercq, F. (2002). Lacan's analytical goal: "Le Sinthome" or the feminine way. In: L.Thurston (Ed.), *Essays on the final Lacan. Re-inventing the symptom.* 59–83. New York: The Other Press.

# Part II

# The Body of Drama

In Part II, the focus turns to Beckett and Artaud. The opening chapter on each author introduces their distinctive aesthetic of the body, showing, in general terms, how their work illuminates mind–body tensions central to the book's argument. The following chapters analyse a key theatrical work by each author, examining how specific performances engage these orientations with the spectator.

DOI: 10.4324/9781003509622-6

Chapter 4

# The Aesthetic of Debility in Beckett's Theatre

The previous chapters posited the body as a question and a traumatic remainder within language, covered by a fantasy construct that shields us from the alienation and trauma at the heart of embodiment. Mind–body narratives are seductive in that they provide meaning to what is fundamentally a hole in sense. One way to challenge them is to identify how ideals of the normal body function to cover the endemic lack of being in subjectivity. This chapter explores how Samuel Beckett's work directly confronts this lack in being, through the ubiquitous figure of the non-normative body, the body that does not conform to a fantasy of the normal. That the body is such a central figure in the lives of his 'characters' defines the somatopsychic dimension of his work, namely the role of the body in shaping the psyche or subjectivity. Psychosomatic perspectives of mind–body relations often deny the ontological instability of the body as an agent of psychical change. One of the ways Beckett's drama challenges normative narratives is not simply through a representation of non-normative or non-conforming bodies but through what is, in essence, an aesthetic of impairment and debility. The pervasiveness of the image of debility or corporeal struggle in Beckett's works implies an underlying orientation in art that premises a form of failure, a non-rapport, at its heart, rather than covering over the cracks in the fantasy of the normal. The difference between a representation and an aesthetic is one of intensity or orientation; a representation may be discrete and intentional, whereas an aesthetic, as a recurring motif or stylistic tendency, is possibly driven by the force of the author's unconscious fantasy. In other words, a particular aesthetic, such as one of failure in Beckett's oeuvre, may serve a structural purpose within an author's subjective economy and feature as a recurring orientation in their work. In using the word orientation, I wish to imply two functions of the term within the context of dramatic works: the orientation of the subject vis-à-vis the object a within the formula for fantasy (the relationship to the Other) on the part of the author and the resulting orientation of the question of meaning within the dramatic work. Orientation is more of a phenomenological term than the more typical psychoanalytic concept of subject position, but it is this within-the-world-aspect I

DOI: 10.4324/9781003509622-7

wish to invoke, most notably in the context of a tangible artwork. While this chapter focuses on a general discussion of the aesthetic of the debilitated body in Beckett's work, the next chapter will use one of his plays, *Endgame*, as a phenomenological case study.

## Debility vs Disability

While I begin by emphasising the term debility, the argument will open onto a discussion of disability as a tangential theme, both represented in and read into Beckett's work. We will see the nuances of these terms subsequently but by focusing more on debility as the driving force of Beckett's aesthetic, I wish to provoke more of an essential engagement with the body as a source of potential decomposition, a site of failure and loss rather than a concrete presentation of an already existing or socio-political signified state, such as disability. This is probably a contentious issue, and it is important to recognise that a distinction between debility and disability has already been made in disability studies by scholars such as Jasbir Puar and Julie Livingston (2005), whose work centres on the socio-political context of debility. According to Puar (2017), the distinction has a temporal and political dimension, with a specificity that affects those in the Global South: "I contend that the term 'debilitation' is distinct from the term 'disablement' because it foregrounds the slow wearing down of populations instead of the event of becoming disabled" (pp. xiii, ix). In this context, however, I wish to use debility not as a political term but as a signifier of suffering and limitation as they relate to the body, as I feel it is less socio-politically inflected than disability. Although debility is certainly a function of disability, depending on the situation or condition, its meaning cannot be collapsed with it. Not all people with disabilities are debilitated, and would certainly not identify that way, for example. However, many people who suffer debilitation, fatigue, innervation, weakness, and malaise as a cause of physical malfunction may identify as disabled. For my purposes in exploring Beckett's work, debility and its negative connotations of failure at an organic level, or where the will or desire is at odds with the limits of the body, provide more of an accurate appraisal of what I feel is going on, to put it in these terms, with the images of the fragmented, ageing, and decrepit characters that populate his texts and drama. Indeed, failure is a theme that I wish to invoke intersectionally in this chapter, failure as conjured within the images and linguistic descriptions of debility in Beckett's works, failure as it relates to a trauma situated within embodiment, to something not working out at the level of the Real that drives our impetus to speak and create within the symbolic, and as an existential driving force that Beckett saw as related to the creative act and the plight of language as expressive of subjectivity.

While linking failure with Beckett's work is nothing new, as Oliver Wallis (2022) examines in an article concerning how the circulation of the phrase from *Worstward Ho,* "Fail again. Fail better" has become indelibly embedded and resignified within popular culture, examining failure as a function of the aesthetic of the body and a signifier of the body's place within subjectivity is potentially provocative and productive of novel associations and perspectives. Although using words such as debility and failure dredge up negative connotations, such as inability, not-doing, inertia, and non-desirability, I feel this potential negativity, with the emphasis on potential, is helpful in exploring narratives and affective states of the body–mind connection in Beckett's work and beyond. We know how the negative and variations of the nothing are the signature of Beckett, so it is not a far cry to consider that this negativity or the drive to uncover the nothingness of being is also written on the body in some way, or that the body features in Beckett's project of subtraction and 'unwording'. Think, for example, of the enclosed world of the body in *Malone Dies* and the varying descriptions of effort and movement required to pick something up with his stick, his physical autonomy restricted to the most minor of tasks, and his environment pared back to that of memory and internal narrative, which is so often a feature of Beckettian characters. When the world is pared down to the body through debility, and this may include states of severe pain (as Elaine Scarry [1985] in *The Body in Pain* contextualises pain as the unmaking of the world), what becomes of ourselves, our memories, our being? To put it simply, an aesthetic of debility accounts for failure as a necessary or ontological component of embodiment. In thinking this way, I am inspired by the queering of failure in works such as Halberstam's *Queer Art of Failure* (2011), where sites of undoing, unbecoming, forgetting, and marginal spaces of knowledge spark modes for thinking differently and where failure and losing are explored as resistance to the toxic positivity adhering to the impetus to achieve and succeed endemic to neoliberal culture. Similarly, Lisa Diedrich's (2005) work on heroic illness narratives and what she calls an ethics of failure[1] as a counterpoint to the injunctions and signifiers often imposed on people who are ill to ultimately overcome their illness through positivity and 'fighting a worthy battle' is in the background of my reading of failure as a motif and an ethical possibility in Beckett's work. When it comes to failure, I think it is important to let it speak for itself as an analogy for the disintegration it may represent. To be blunt, not to sugarcoat it and formulate rehabilitative interpretations that dilute the potential affects/effects it generates.

Indeed, if we were to coin a phrase for the ethical import of Beckett's work, it could also be an ethics of failure, where the worldview of the writer is one in which all characters are anti-heroes, struggling against the erosions of conventional meaning and the vagaries of beleaguered selfhood in sometimes menacing and always sparse environments; there are no 'winners' in the crude, populist sense of attaining or displaying cultural achievement, prowess, and productivity. Again, the relationship between failure and ethics in Beckett's aesthetic is a well-trodden path in the literature, as scholars such as Rabaté and Tereszewski in *The Aesthetics of Failure* (2013) have given voice to. Both critics emphasise the opportunity for a radical encounter with alterity that arises from the theme of the failure of expression, or the drive to say the ontologies of the nothing so endemic to Beckett's texts and drama. Rabaté refers to this ethical momentum as the "ethics of nonrelation", a phrase with distinct Lacanian echoes of "there is no sexual relation". That is, apart from the more complex ramifications of this statement within the field of sexuality, we can say that in a Lacanian sense, there is always a degree of non-rapport for the human subject within the context of human relationships and object relating; communication falls short of receptive complementarity, and subject and object do not cohere neatly and reciprocally. As Rabaté puts it, "The key term nonrelation destroys from the outset the humanistic illusion that we are alike, or that human reciprocity should be taken as a given. On the contrary, it is because we are all infinitely different that a true rapport can be posited" (2016, p. 91). Rabaté's ethics of the nonrelation is also based on what he calls Beckett's commitment to an art of poverty, influenced by the ethical philosophy of the occasionalist Geulincx, an aesthetic characterised by the dehiscence of the self, humility, and the mysteries of the will. When it comes to Beckett's orientation to the body, particularly the impaired body, the philosophy of Geulincx, as a backdrop to the motifs of bodily immobility, inertia, passivity, and powerlessness in Beckett's drama, is fascinating and enlightening. I will return to this point later. For now, let us look at Beckett's own words on the subject of art, expression, failure, and the obligation to create, which feature strongly in critiques of the ethical inflexions of his aesthetic.

In the following passage, taken from the three dialogues with George Duthuit in which he expresses his views on the visual arts, and speaking of the Dutch painter Bram van Velde, Beckett refers to the possibility of a new type of relation borne of failure, and affirms that to be an artist is to fail, even to be driven to fail and that this is the impossible but necessary obligation of the creative act:

> My case, since I am in the dock, is that Van Velde is the first to desist from this aestheticized automatism, the first to admit that to be an artist is to fail, as no other dare fail, that failure is his world and the shrink from it desertion, art and craft, good housekeeping, living. No, no allow me to expire. I know that all that is required now, in order to bring even this horrible matter to an acceptable conclusion, is to make of this submission, this admonition, this fidelity to failure, a new occasion, a new form of relation, and of the act which, unable to act, obliged to act, he makes, an expressive act, even if only of itself, of the impossibility, of its obligation.
>
> (quoted in Cohn, *Disjecta Membra*, 1984)

This passage is highly revealing of the paradoxes inherent in Beckett's work regarding the predicament of his characters or ghostly apparitions and their relation to expression, speech, and communication. As the voice in *The Unnamable* exhibits, there are no words with which to express the essence of the subject or the personal pronoun, no words that can bring silence to the ravings and vacillations of memory and internal narrative and yet the 'I' is compelled to express, to go on speaking, even as words exhaust themselves in the process. Ultimately, the I, that shifter of the precarious personal pronoun, *fails* to ever utter a word that can capture and put an end to the process of speaking either internally or to another. Speech is interminable as long as the subject lives, yet this ongoingness reveals a fissure between subject and other. The subject/object relationship of speaker and addressee is not neatly contained within the play of signifier and signified, certainly not as the internal voice of speech displays. There is an excess to the act of speaking, what Lacan calls jouissance, an enjoyment beyond what is said, that is revealed in Beckett's plays and prose. This excess exists in the very enunciation of emitting words, regardless of the "neatness of identifications" (Beckett, 1984) proffered by the seductions of meaning. However, the failure of language to say the self or identify an essence as captured within *The Unnamable* is ontologically paradoxical as Rabaté explains, "if language fails to capture the speaker's singularity, it also grants him an existence—understood as an ecstatic being of nonbeing—but only as long as he speaks" (Rabaté, 2016, p. 44). The fact that language is imbued with failure, in terms of ever catching a linguistic hold of this elusive I, or achieving a silence of being, a being that is tied to language, at least in the context of *The Unnamable*, allows a spotlight to shine on the gap or discord between the ego represented by the personal pronoun and the subject of the unconscious. From a Lacanian point of view, the I who speaks is not the same entity as the subject of the unconscious; as we have seen in the context of alienation, meaning and being are in opposing circles. The enunciating subject and the subject of the enunciation are not the same thing. We find ourselves navigating complex terrain on what exactly constitutes the nature of being, within Lacan's works and Beckett's but also in the interstices of the dialogue of this book. This complexity is somehow implicated through the Beckettian motif of failure as the obligation to express, through a speaking entity that fails to express adequately, within an embodied form that often staggers and stutters (Deleuze, 1998). If form is content and content is form, as often is the case with Beckettian drama, Beckett's debilitated or truncated bodies may literally materialise something difficult or impossible to say in language that is related to the very limits of language and expressibility—the trauma of the failure of the body at the material level and the failure of language to say a body or to say what a body is in its entirety. But how can we say that Beckett's bodies fail or that failure is inherent to embodiment, let alone say that this failure can be traumatic? We do not need to invoke anything non-normative to speak of failure as immanent to our corporality and to the functioning of organs and component parts; as Damasio (2021) says, no amount of free will can prevent the inevitable end to our existence or, as he puts it, "the destiny your genome has set for you".

## Not Failing Better

As a mortal substance, the human body is destined to fail, and it ultimately abandons us to death with the final cessation of breath. An entropic force underpins corporeal existence and, indeed, perhaps the whole universe itself. The body we possess does not always (or ever) match up to our expectations of it; it can falter, interrupt us through pain, illness, fall prey to accidents, disobey our will, and eventually, we will die as a result of its finite condition. Failure is not just a noun but can also be an affect, a felt sense, a signifier for psychic and emotional states and connotes aspects of the subjective experience of acquiring damage to the body. The limitations induced by disease, including sensations of physical pain, can feel like a rupture at the level of the organism—something is not working within the body or has failed to function. We may intend to move, but the body does not obey our will. The relationship between the will and bodily impairment as an affect of failure is illustrated in the title of Lisa I. Iezzoni's research on mobility problems in *When Walking Fails* (2003). The following passage gives voice to this feeling:

> Some people refer to their bodies in the third person, as does Sally Ann Jones: "I say to my feet, 'Move, dammit!' And they say, 'No. We are on strike.' … It's almost like your brain is saying, 'Do something! Do something!' And your body is not responding. In my mind, I'm doing something, but in reality, my limbs are not moving.
>
> (2003, p. 70)

Furthermore, although certain situations bring a sense of failure into stark relief, such as sudden paralysis or physical immobilisation caused by pain, there is a failure (at the level of the body and representation) that also accompanies all states of embodiment. There is always a gap between the body (and indeed the organism) as we imagine it to be and that which it 'is' concerning ourselves and other embodied subjects. We can revisit the mirror stage we examined in the previous chapter and how we identify with, or incorporate, an inaccurate reflection of who we are as a bodily entity. The image of the body is introjected as the basis of the ego, the correlate of the one who says 'I'. In a sense, we fail to truly see ourselves as we really are, largely because this cannot be captured in the specular image. What is also not captured in real time in the specular image is the process of change we undergo throughout life, a change that feels like loss. As Hamm in *Endgame* says: "But we breathe, we change! We lose our hair, our teeth! Our bloom! Our ideals!" (Beckett, 1958/2006, p. 97). The slow encroachment of debility with ageing (as it happens for many, more suddenly for others in the case of certain disabilities) is not a reality lauded or desired by neoliberal culture and is a spectre of the imagos of the autonomous, self-supporting, productive, youthful, and successful individual that haunt the imagistic objects of popular culture. Never is this idea of declining or failing[2] embodiment more clearly represented than in Samuel Beckett's oeuvre, where across the span of his work from prose to drama, we encounter 'characters' with bodies that stagger, limp, struggle, crawl, remain fixed in position, are trapped in some way or alone in the dark, and are reduced to fragments or part-objects, such as Mouth in *Not I* (1972), the bodiless heads of *Play* (1963) and Nell and Nag in the dustbins of *Endgame* (1958). In *Happy Days* (1961), the body is subject to the encroachment of the environment as the sand increasingly envelops the seemingly nonchalant Winnie. In this instance, the environment may serve as a visual metaphor for the existential constraints of the subject, hemmed in by ever-decreasing circles of possibility as time passes. Winnie's seeming indifference to the suffocating sand further emphasises the act's existential quality. The ubiquity of these immobilised or physically restricted characters is striking and leads to the consideration that, for Beckett, the constrained body serves as a metaphor for unnameable or ineffable psychic states. As Siobhan Purcell (2018) argues: "States of paralysis and immobility are not simply sites of inertia but are instead recast by Beckett as pared down moments of reflection on the will, the wish, and on external pressures" (p. 190). In other words, the restricted body gives form to the affective or psychical experience of other, less tangible subjective restrictions. That being said, we could also say that the restricted body of Beckett's drama gives materiality to an ethereal dimension of mind, an aspect of psychic reality that feels 'disabled' or constrained by the physical frame of embodiment. As I have said, disability can involve feelings of failure, limitation, and restriction and can be an apt description of a feeling of psychic impotence.

The sheer ubiquity of what could be called the disabled or incapacitated body in Beckett's work is intriguing, although, as we shall see, we have to be careful with these definitions so as to avoid reducing the complexity of form to preformulated signifiers or words with associations that tame or pigeonhole the unruliness of these Beckettian metaphors. The pervasiveness of the 'disabled body' in Beckett's drama and prose has lent itself to much recent interrogation as to the usefulness of applying a disability-orientated theoretical lens to his failing bodies. While certainly not conforming to the medical model of disability—in Beckett's work, disability is not presented as something to be cured (as a medical or even tragic phenomenon), but rather as essential to the existential experience of life and the characterisation of his protagonists—the representation is far from the social model. Bodily ailments and physical impositions are so frequent that it suggests that considering the human subject as ideal or grandiose regarding the manifestation of embodiment would be a farce. A great example of this is found in the novel *Watt* (1953), in which several generations of the Lynch family are, one after the other, afflicted in every way imaginable with disease and physical misfortune, and the reader (this reader) cannot help but laugh at such depictions. While it may be tempting to interpret the presence of lameness, immobility, blindness, and a general leaning towards corporeal imperfection as markers of a disability-orientated perspective in the positivistic sense, that is, as bringing something to light that had remained heretofore hidden, these interpretations may lose something of the subversive potential of these bodily signs and symptoms. As Hannah Simpson points out, "Beckett's plays are not straightforwardly 'activist' disability texts in any uplifting or politically correct way. These are playscripts which deploy the impaired or unexpectedly functioning body as a central element of their unsettling aesthetic and affective effect" (Simpson, 2002, p. 208). Simpson's study of Beckett's work examines how plays such as *Not I, Endgame*, and *Waiting for Godot* have been performed by self-identified disabled actors, and the nuances of bodily integrity or ontological verisimilitude they provoke. Often, the actors have identified the nuances or particularities of their own disability/impairment or bodily difference within the language, actions, and bodily specificities of the 'characters', figures, or ghostly apparitions that populate the sparse Beckettian landscape.

## Body–Mind Relations

Many of Beckett's works lend themselves at least partially to interpretations or speculations that place the brain's relation to physical disease/impairment at the centre of the unfolding spectacle or narrative. The play *Not I*, for example, has been performed by performer and activist Jess Thom, who has Tourette syndrome and relates to Mouth's logorrhoeic outpourings as the involuntary, neurological tics associated with the condition. As she said in a *Guardian* interview, "I really identify Mouth as a neurodiverse character and feel that hers is—in part—my story to tell" (2017, 13 August). As critics such as Rina Kim and Lois Oppenheim have argued through a neuroscientific lens, Beckett had a keen interest in the brain and in his own psychosomatic or somatopsychic symptomatology, which compelled him to read prominent works on the brain and to seek out psychoanalysis with Wilfred Bion. Apart from being interested in the source of his own physiological symptoms, what I find compelling is what Rina refers to as Beckett's somatosensory interest in the synaptic gaps of the brain, or to put this in dangerously simple language, where the brain impacts the body (and thus the mind, from Damasio's neuroscientific perspective) in an unconscious way. Furthermore, Beckett's interest in the mind–body problem and the very evident philosophical influences and inclinations regarding this rapport/non-rapport in his work are intriguing. The Cartesian resonances of his work are well flagged, and indeed, Beckett's first published poem, *Whoroscope* (1930), displays a keen interest in the contentious but hugely influential philosopher. In this poem, a grumpy René Descartes awaits the serving of an extremely mature egg. However, while Beckett's work sometimes displays a Cartesian approach to the experience of embodiment (as linguistically exemplified by specific passages in *Murphy* where a clear split is expressed between psyche and soma), and potentially revealed imagistically through the truncation of heads without bodies (in *Play, Not I* and *The Unnamable*), where the mind raves on without a functioning body attached, it cannot be reduced to a Cartesian reading, particularly as the so-called rational subject of the cogito is so frequently subverted as unknowing and inherently unreliable. In fact, as Anthony Uhlmann (2006) argues in an annotated volume of Geulincx's *Ethics* (p. 306), the cogito that is described in *The Unnamable* is more of a Geulincxian cogito than a Cartesian one, as it leads to an understanding that one knows nothing, rather than building a solid foundation from which to know the world. Geulincx's ethical philosophy is centred on the principle of humility, which he calls "not caring about oneself" or abandoning oneself to go to or be with God. As mentioned earlier, Beckett had a keen interest in Geulincx's ethics, and his transcriptions and notes on the treatise are of great importance for tracing the mind–body context and, perhaps, the negations of the pursuit of happiness in his work. For Geulincx, the cause of the movements of the body and the workings of the organs cannot be known by us directly; they can only be occasioned by God, and we need to surrender or abandon ourselves to the not-knowing. The following passage is taken from the annotated ethics and illustrates Geulincx's perspective on God as a source of knowledge or cause concerning the physical organs:

> Once we have learned from inspection of ourselves which things are ours and which are God's, and in particular, that we do not create the motion of our organs, that the eye essentially brings nothing to seeing, that the world cannot of its own accord reveal itself to our gaze, and that all these things are done by the ineffable power of someone else; once, I say, we have come to see ourselves as we really are through inspecting these and suchlike things, the vulgar call us insane, holding that this business of self-inspection leads to stark raving madness, not to wisdom.
>
> (Guelincx, 2006, p. xi)

Guelincx's perspective on movement and the will is interesting in relation to the motifs of failure, will, and debility in Beckett's aesthetics, and it will allow for a deeper exploration of disability as a representation of contingency in his work. One of the reasons I find this connection so intriguing is that it allows for a reading of disability that falls outside certain narratives of representation and can lead us toward the aesthetic of debility, which opens up the question of being. In other words, the figures of debility (or disability, as a reading we may place on these figures) encompass philosophical reflections on the roles of autonomy, causation, humility, and the limits of knowledge and possibility. Indeed, the experience of disability often leads to a consideration of these very questions. For example, a person may grapple with the very essence of what constitutes being when the external façade of the imaginary body is challenged by disease or functional alteration. It has been said that Beckett may have had a disability, in terms of the symptoms he suffered both physically and mentally. Whether this is relevant or not is questionable, but certainly, Beckett's interest in the mind–body relation was not simply philosophical but also personal (although of course one often inspires or provokes the other), and he may well have experienced a sense of failure concerning his own will and the symptoms he suffered from in his body. As Kim says:

> While Beckett seemed to have been interested in the Cartesian split even before he undertook psychoanalytic therapy sessions with Wilfred Bion from 1933 to 1935, the idea of psychosomatic origins for mental distress also seemed to impel him to explore the relation between the mind and the body, their close link on the one hand and their failure to interact on the other, particularly in the context of the body disobeying one's own will.
>
> (Kim, 2016, p. 153)

Kim has focused on something critically important in the above quote: the body and mind are not mutually reciprocal or complementary entities, and failure can be a feature of our experience of the will or desire as it relates to matters of the body. We saw in the above example regarding walking that, depending on circumstances, physical condition, or disability, walking or movement may fail to occur even when we desire or will it to happen. This experience can be one of immense frustration, anxiety, and loss, and poses a challenge to an individual's sense of bodily integrity and sense of self. If we think of particular diseases that cause disruptions to body movement or feeling in profound ways (and there are so many, so not mentioning them does not preclude them), such as motor neurone disease, multiple sclerosis, myalgic encephalomyelitis, and cancer, at moments or phases where the disease has the upper hand, the will, although it does have a place in living with the disease, cannot overturn the physiological damage caused by the disease. I do not want to imply that psychological states do not play a role in disease/illness but I want to underline the very common reality that the effects of these diseases often feel like a failure at the level of desire and the will. In other words, I wish to infer a relation from the somatopsychic rather than the psychosomatic angle, and to query the role of changes in body state across a range of subjective parameters, including emotional, psychological, and effects on the unconscious. There has been a strong overhang historically and culturally in our psyches of the idea that illness/disability is equated with sin or a moral failing at some level. However, I think this overhang of societal and self-blame toward bodily difference, or dysfunction, is a little different, though somewhat connected to the affectual state of being unable to will the body into action. For example, it appears to be commonplace among people with illness/disabilities to find internal psychological reasons for why aspects of the body may have failed/be failing to operate as usual or to account for fluctuations in the course of a physical condition/illness. This is in part a defensive response to the unknown and the feeling of being out of control, and it may be comforting to think that there is something we can do to put things 'right'. Freud refers to this kind of superego condemnation in *Civilisation and Its Discontents* (1930), regarding the personal interpretations we may give to negative or regrettable acts of fate. The fact that we can infer from Beckett's work an interest in the very failure of the will to act on the body, or the question of their connectivity, or indeed lack of connectivity, as well as the environmental restrictions imposed on bodies, lends itself to considering the somatopsychic implications of states of confinement, incarceration, restriction, and torture. We can note that the latter can all be deemed negative or painful scenarios, in which we may encounter the limits of what a human being can endure, suffer, or tolerate. It is also obvious that Beckett is interested in mining the limits of existence, an existence supported by the pillars of language and the materiality of the flesh. This courting of the limit, how far the subject can go before it disappears into the void beyond language, could also be driving the aesthetic of debility in both its imagistic production on stage and linguistic description in written texts. To state the question simply again, how do changes in the body state or what Damasio refers to as background bodily feeling alter the mind, the memory, the internal body image we have of ourselves and the sense of the one who says I? Another way of thinking about this is from the perspective of unconscious desire in Lacanian psychoanalysis—how is desire implicated when something goes wrong or fails to work at the level of the body? A key point to make here is not that Beckett provides the answers to these questions through his drama or prose, but that an accent is placed on the body as ontologically imperfect, and that the relation between psyche and soma is problematised rather than simplified.

Similarly, Oppenheim makes the point that although Beckett is deeply interested in the body-mind connection (psyche/soma), it has not received much exploration in critical research (2005, p. 71). She also makes a neuroscientific argument for the homeostatic role that the act of creativity performs for Beckett and his endless projections and figurations of a self that is unstable and dissolving between inside and outside. My question is not simply why this somatopsychic emphasis exists in Beckett's work, although I am intrigued by what motivates (consciously or unconsciously) the aesthetic of debility or failure, but what phenomenological value we can infer from a somatosensory perspective in approaching his work. In other words, what makes these depictions so relatable, and why do they resonate so much with the Beckettian-orientated viewer/reader? Has Beckett really captured something of the subjective essence of corporeal existence, in Damasio's or Solms's terms, what it really *feels* like to be or to have a body, or do we have yet another imaginary veil of the body, another image in a mis-en-abyme of images, forever perpetuating meconnaisance? To be more precise, what aspect of subjectivity is Beckett capturing through the aesthetic of the impaired body? While we could say that on the whole, Beckett's oeuvre is not specifically about disability in a narrative sense, in other words, it does not actively support or dispel a view of either the social or medical model of disability,[3] and his characters do not generally reveal their feelings about their ailments, his work nonetheless provides increasingly fertile ground for critique and investigation on the terrain of the non-normative, in general, but also as it concerns disability/impairment. As I said earlier, failure is a feature of the impaired body in Beckett's drama, as a symbol of something ineffable about being, and also as a signifier of the existential condition of humanity per se. In fact, it might be more accurate to say that being itself is ineffable, and this is what Beckett circles through words with no end and bodies that fail. Being cannot be said; it can only be approached through a process of subtraction or negation, where negation does not nullify existence but circumscribes an essential no-body, the subject of the unconscious. As the following words from Tereszewski regarding Beckett's relationship to nothing brilliantly illustrate:

> This neutrality serves the purpose of allowing the hypostatic nothingness to speak. However, in a Heideggerian turn, what is ultimately elevated by means of negation of being is being itself. Being is resuscitated by its negation.
>
> (2013, p. 40)

I'll admit I'm not Heideggerian in my reading of this quote, but I think there is also a Lacanian twist here. As Lacan argues in Seminar IX, *Identification*, negation is at the heart of the birth of the subject, with -1 being the designation of this elusive entity, and the signifier only becoming a signifier through a form of effacement of a trace. The signifier is what remains after the negation of an original mark, the unary trait, that serves as a point of identification for the subject. In an almost chiasmatic process, the signifier and the subject engender each other:

> The neurotic does not know, and with good reason, that it is *qua* subject that he has fomented the following: the advent of the signifier in so far as the signifier is the principal effacing of the thing, that it is he, the subject who by effacing all the traits of the thing, makes the signifier.
>
> (Lacan, 1961, Session XIII, 14 March 1962, p. 129)

Let's now take into account what I discussed in Chapter 3 about the discord between the subject of the unconscious and the body. The being of the subject exists as a function of the signifier, but the signifier, to a certain extent, transcends the physical body, while also causing a traumatic inscription on the flesh. Words 'matter' literally and yet have a life of their own beyond the body. Beckett frequently captures this non-coincidence between body and language, in which memory and narrative operate without a functioning body. Even if we could say that the vision of life portrayed doesn't make logical sense, such as a head talking in a jar, when in reality, without a body, we could not talk, a discord or aporia of being is represented through this organic impossibility. We can hear this aporia in the following words from *Worstward Ho:* "Say a body. Where none. No mind. Where none. That at least. A place. Where none. For the body" (Beckett, 1989, p. 101). The body itself is a question and not something that can be readily identified, at least in language, or by invoking the presence of the physical flesh as a definitive anchor of being. At least not as an either/or of this equation. The body has being in both words and flesh, it is a hybrid object, something spoken in absentia and felt viscerally in the shadows of silence. Words don't match the affectual realm, but both exist as markers of the subject's relation to the body, a relation that has a discordant dimension. I realise what I am describing here is abstract and precariously Cartesian, but perhaps we are in Cartesian affectual waters (rather than actual) when we speak of being. That is, to speak of being is to engender a division inherent to language. Language cannot say the all of being—a portion of it remains opaque. While Lacan was always at pains to overturn Descartes' cogito and the privileging of thought as ontological certainty, the discrepancy between the body and the mind or between the subject and the unconscious has not been accounted for. I argue that this discrepancy is exactly what Beckett captures in the discordant spectacles of alienated subjects whose bodies don't match up with the outpourings of the mind. Another way of saying it is that disability or debility is a fantasised means of accessing being through a reduction of all exterior distractions, where the world is reduced to the bare boards of a minimalist interior. Enter *Endgame*, one of Beckett's bleakest plays, but the one he said he disliked the least.

## Notes

1 The ethics of failure is a term Deidrich takes from Jacqueline Rose and then applies to the work of Jackie Stacey and Gillian Rose in books on their experience of ovarian cancer. She describes an ethics of failure as "an ethics that emerges out of the experience of failure and in these cases the failure of the body, of conventional and alternative medicine, and of language. Such an ethics, which draws on both feminist and postmodern formulations of bioethics, challenges autonomy as the primary aim of bioethics, as well as the heroic narratives that limit other ethical formulations that might emerge out of the experience of illness" (2005, p. 135).

2 I am aware of the problematic and potentially stigmatising connotations of connecting the word failure with debility/disability/ illness but the use is deliberate and reflective both of my personal experience and what I feel to be pertinent in the accent Beckett places on these bodies. The body does not always obey our will and ultimately it can gain the upper hand in our destiny, regardless of our desires. The relation between desire and movement or desire and physical limitation is extremely complex, particularly if we take desire to be unconscious as any use of the term in this book certainly does. Although self-referring to personal experience as a phenomenological and defensive position may be hackneyed in academic discourse, I feel it is relevant to highlight the necessary invocation of the subjective feeling of pain, illness, disability, limitation, and ultimately the parameters of embodiment per se.

3 The discussion of the social model vs the medical model of disability refers to the longstanding critique of the medical model that implies that disability is a deficit in the individual. The social model by contrast argues that disability is a function of society; it is society and the lack of support offered that cause a person to be disabled.

## References


Adorno, T. & Jones, M.T. (1982). Trying to understand *Endgame. New German Critique*, 26, 119–150.

Beckett, S. (1958). *Endgame.* Grove Press.

Beckett, S. (1984). Three dialogues. In R. Cohn (Ed.), *Disjecta membra: Miscellaneous writings and a dramatic fragment by Samuel Beckett.* Grove Press.

Beckett, S. (1989). *Nohow On: Company, Ill Seen Ill Said, and Worstward Ho.* Grove Press.

Damasio, A. (2021). *Feeling and knowing.* YouTube video: Harvard Book Store. https://www.youtube.com/watch?v=A_BX5n6CWlg.

Deleuze, G. (1998). He stuttered. In *Essays critical and clinical* (D. W. Smith & M. A. Greco, Transl., pp. 107–114). Verso.

Diedrich, L. (2005). A bioethics of failure: Antiheroic cancer narratives in *Ethics of the body: Postconventional challenges* (eds) M. Shildrick and R. Mykitiuk. Cambridge/London/Massachusetts: The MIT Press.

Geulincx, A. (2006). *Ethics: With Samuel Beckett's notes* (M. Wilson, Transl.; H. van Ruler, A. Uhlmann, & M. Wilson, Eds.). Leiden: Brill Academic Publishers. (Original work published in Latin as *De virtute et primis eius proprietatibus*)

Halberstam, J. (2011). *The queer art of failure.* Duke University Press.

Iezzoni, L. (2003). *When walking fails: Mobility problems of adults with chronic conditions.* University of California Press.

Kim, R (2016). [G]azing into the synaptic chasm": the brain in Beckett's writing. *Journal of Medical Humanities.* 37 (2), 149–160.

Kumar, K.J. (1997). The chess metaphor in Samuel Beckett's *Endgame. Modern Drama.* 40 (4), 540–552.

Lacan, J. (1961–1962). *The seminar of Jacques Lacan. Book IX, Identification.* Transl. C. Gallagher. Unpublished

Mansell, T. (2007). Hard-to-hear music in Endgame. In (eds) Mark S. Byron & Michael J. Mayer, *Samuel Beckett's Endgame.* Amsterdam & New York: Rodopi.

Oppenheim, L. (2005). *A curious intimacy: Art and psychoanalysis.* London: Routledge.

Puar, J. K. (2017). *The right to maim: Debility/capacity/disability*. Duke University Press.

Purcell, S. (2018). *Extraordinary debilities: Disability in the works of Samuel Beckett*. Unpublished PhD Thesis NUIG: Galway.

Rabaté, J.M. (2016). *Think, Pig! Beckett at the limit of the human*. New York: Fordham University Press.

Scarry, E. (1985). *The body in pain: The making and unmaking of the world*. Oxford University Press.

Simpson, H. (2022). *Samuel Beckett and disability performance*. Palgrave Macmillan.

Tereszewski, M. (2013). *The aesthetics of failure: Inexpressibility in Samuel Beckett's Fiction*. Cambridge Scholars Publishing.

Thom, J. (2017). Interview with Jess Thom: 'I don't suppress my tics – it's definitely Beckett with biscuits'. *The Guardian* newspaper online. https://www.theguardian.com/stage/2017/aug/13/jess-thom-touretteshero-samuel-beckett-not-i-edinburgh-fringe-festival.

Wallis. O. (2022). The allure of "fail better": Uses of Beckett's modernist cliché. *College Literature*, 49 (1), 26–52.

Chapter 5

# "Something is Taking its Course"

## Endgame's Chronic Bodies

*Endgame* is one of Beckett's most well-known, hermeneutically intransigent, and notoriously desolate plays. From the outset, the opening emits a fatal tone, and we are drawn into a scene where time and existence may be drawing to a close, yet without an obvious cause. It is not certain what is happening, but "something is taking its course" and "nearly finished". Clov's opening lines, reminiscent of the crucifixion, set the apocalyptic tone: "Finished, it's finished, nearly finished, it must be nearly finished" (1958/2006, p. 93). We are immediately alerted to the presence of suffering and to the desire for it to end.

### A Moribund World

The play begins with the unveiling of inanimate objects; there is a stillness, a corpse-like feel to the objects on stage. Hamm is covered by a sheet and motionless in an armchair. A sheet also covers both dustbins that are situated behind Hamm. Clov appears and shuffles around the room, removing the sheets and opening the blinds, laughing curiously and somewhat hysterically at each unveiling. There is no marker of standard chronological time; the time is 'zero', signifying a space outside the usual markers of everyday temporality. We are in no man's land. If the time is zero, the ambience is akin to ground zero, a location directly impacted by a hostile threat. As Hamm exclaims, "Outside of here it's death" (1958/2006, p. 96).

The characters of *Endgame* seem, to a great degree, powerless, each in their own way, to alter the environment in which they find themselves. Hamm, Clov, Nell, and Nagg are enclosed in a sparse, minimally furnished room, all compromised by physical restrictions and tied to each other like a set of mutually dependent entities. Nell and Nagg are trapped in dustbins and at the mercy of their son Hamm, who is blind and confined to a chair.[1] The only room in the one-act play is dark and shabby, minimalist and sparse, dislocated from anywhere familiar and situated in an unknown territory. This adds to the intimation of an impending checkmate in the play; the environment of the characters is closing in on them, and they may be encountering

DOI: 10.4324/9781003509622-8

the last few moves available to them vis-à-vis existence itself, just as in the closing stages of a game of chess when few pieces remain on the board. Hamm's initial words, "Me… to play" (p. 93), mark the opening of an implied game, the potentiality of making a move. While *Endgame* intrinsically resists interpretation, the chess metaphor has featured prominently in criticism and is a motif in Beckett's work. According to Kumar, it "functions as a unifying element" of various symbols in the play and "presents the existential angst of man through the uncertainty and unpredictability of the last phase of a game of chess" (1997, p. 540). While I disagree that *Endgame* can be read in any unifying way, it is a play certainly replete with symbolism and existential angst. This existential angst is reflected in the bleak environment of *Endgame*, the linguistic repetitions of things running out or ceasing to exist, and is a function of the staging of bodies that reveal the inherent mortality of the human being. Hamm's paralytic confinement causes him to be moved (pushed by Clov) around the stage as a chess piece would be around a board. He is both king of his surroundings, giving orders and commanding moves, yet a passive recipient of what is taking its course in the environment. Without any obvious cause for the events, nature, the dominant overseer, appears to be driving events. Yet, even nature, as the support for life, is running out. Clov: "There's no more nature. Hamm: No more nature! You exaggerate" (1958/2006 p. 97). An air of finality hangs over the dialogue and the characters' actions, and a shadow of futility is cast over all. However, this gloomy atmosphere is cut through with a dark humour inherent to this absurdist situation, as in Hamm and Clov's master-slave dynamic, and the bizarre confinement of Hamm's parents to dustbins.

Hamm and Clov are tied together in a quasi-sadomasochistic coupling in which they are dependent on each other for survival. Hamm appears to control Clov, blowing a whistle to call him to attention. In the background, Hamm's decrepit parents take up an uncanny spectral presence, appearing on occasion with ashen white, bedraggled faces. Imprisoned by their dustbins, Nell and Nagg are unable to touch each other beyond their metal enclosures (although they try and fail)—a stark and figural example of the Lacanian non-rapport. Consequently, they are in solitary confinement once the lid is closed and serve as metaphors for aloneness and isolation, "the old folks at home" (Beckett, 1958/2006, p. 96).

As we saw in the previous chapter, Beckett's aesthetic of debility incorporates failure as a gritty motif of the body. In relegating the aged to dustbins, Beckett has aligned the elderly (as symbolic figures of the temporality of the body) with the abject, Kristeva's term (1982) for a state in which the distinction between subject and object is threatened by bodily processes that signify our inherent potential for disintegration and render the symbolic infected by death. The abject is the realm of sensations of disgust, repudiation, and rejection, but it can also be one of fascination. We are often drawn towards our disintegration as subjects or, more specifically, ego-subjects. A dustbin is where we throw discarded and useless waste products, rotting and decaying food, and the remains of our daily lives. As an image or signifier of the abject, the dustbin is a container for the repudiated and disgusting remnants of the flesh. Apart from being emblems of corporeal remnants, Nell and Nag also serve as representations of the remainders of Hamm's life, ghostly figures with a disembodied presence; we only ever see their heads—Nagg refers to his stumps in sawdust as if he has no legs. The body as a totalising image is acutely absent. Metaphorically, Nell and Nagg are like the dying embers of Hamm's imagination or psychic memories, and he can never see them in the flesh, not least as he is also blind. Positioned behind him, they serve as a ghostly chorus, suggesting that these figures are representations in memory, traces of the mother and father he once had. The relationship between Hamm and his parents is not one of tenderness; they irritate him and are nuisances to be kept a lid on. Nagg is the "cursed progenitor", the one who is cursed with having given Hamm life.

Within the dynamics between Hamm and his parents, it could be said that Hamm is punishing them, enacting a revenge fantasy in which he can dominate and control in a way he was powerless to do as a boy. Nagg and Hamm's dialogue reveals aspects of Hamm's interior life. According to Nagg, when Hamm was a baby, he was not listened to; he cried, but there was no response. Nagg's taunting is malicious as he hopes that one day Hamm will need to be listened to, that he will experience what it is like to have that vulnerability. Hamm then shares this resentful tone by telling Clov that one day, he too, might be blind and need help, but there will be nobody there. These fractious relations between Hamm and his father, while exposing the history of a particular relationship, also point to a relational motif in Beckett's work—an absence at the heart of communication where a cry for help cannot be adequately responded to, there is no other that can alleviate the angst of living—"the air is full of our cries" (Beckett, 1953/2006, p. 84). The non-rapport of communication reveals a gap in the symbolic, where the Other (or to whom the cry is addressed) fails to respond adequately to this cry or suffering; Godot never arrives, and night never comes. While the non-response has a specific context in light of attachment, containment, and responses that can alleviate anxiety in a child, its place as a motif serves a more structural and existential function in *Endgame* and Beckett's work. The Other lacks—in Lacanian terms, it is barred, incomplete, divided. Even the toy dog that lacks a leg bears something of this non-rapport of communication. Hamm wishes that the dog would gaze at him in adoration but it duly falls over, without a leg to stand on.

As many factors in the setting of *Endgame* are ambiguous, such as location, time, and meaning, the bodies of the characters are positioned not simply in their infirmity but also as the dislocated objects of a moribund world. Their relative powerlessness and dependence on each other subvert the fantasy of narcissistic mastery pertaining to the imaginary structure of the ego and, by so doing, render the situation darkly comic. In this decaying environment, all the characters experience impairment at a physical level, and there are no ideals of 'healthy', 'happy' embodiment. In its stead, rather than witnessing the fantasy of normality, which is upheld by representations of abled bodies and subtended by heroic narratives and tales of overcoming, we encounter the fantasy of debility, a world where to be is to suffer through the body. As Hannah Simpson (2022) puts it:

> If Beckett's work presents disability as the norm rather than the exception, reflecting the reality that all human bodies deviate from an idealised standard of perfect functioning, and all acquire various impairments over the course of the lives (whether diagnosed as disability, dysfunction, dependency, injury, illness, or old age), in *Endgame* this recognition is underscored with a particularly dark menace rather than a utopian acceptance,
>
> (p. 84).

In *Endgame*, from the spectator's point of view, there is no contrast on stage with any able-bodied character that would give the specular juxtaposition of disability versus the able-bodied. We could say that there is no imaginary point of normative or idealistic ability, no comparison with bodies that 'function' autonomously or independently. In other words, there is no contrast with an image of the 'norm' or an ideal from which these bodies become registered as disabled; they simply exist as is.

## The Fantasy of Debility

In *Endgame*, the aesthetic of debility is pervasive. This aesthetic is pertinent not only to the representation of the body as impaired, restricted, dying, or disabled but also to the intimations of loss and mourning that shadow the objects either mentioned or shown in the play. A fundamental erasure of form is at work, more in a phenomenological outer worldly sense than what occurs in Beckett's later plays and texts, where the modes of artistic production are pared back and where imagination and words are stripped back to their very signifierness. In *Endgame*, this erasure is both visual and linguistic (the characters speak of loss) and is inscribed on the body as signs of life's decay and entropy. The world seems to be closing in on this decrepit room in a godforsaken place; all avenues for escape and relief are running out, including the potential for the body to distract itself from itself through "pain killers", "Turkish delight", or any item of pleasure. While the bodies in *Endgame* could be classified as disabled, this is not a representation of disability that succumbs to narratives of political correctness or tragedy, nor does it challenge negative conceptions of disability, quite possibly the opposite; rather, from the perspective of fantasy, an orientation toward the object a within the unconscious, the impaired bodies of *Endgame* are figures through which to perform a process of subtraction on the self and are more aligned with what I have described in the previous chapter as debilitated. A question could certainly be asked here: why am I calling these bodies debilitated and not disabled? I think they are both; we can't say they are *not* disabled, but it is more useful to consider them as debilitated by the overall aesthetic of the play and perhaps by remembering some of the more political or social associations already made in the previous chapter with this word. Also, I would question whether disability, per se, was even on Beckett's mind with these representations, which is not to say that it wasn't there unconsciously. That is, I think, within the context of *Endgame*—its numerous references, either directly or obliquely, to emptiness, barrenness, a void, a nullity, zero—the bodies are an extension of this inexorable uncovering of nothing. I will return to this idea in the final part of this chapter when I discuss the pain of existence as that state of being to which the play is edging towards. That disability is more in line here with debility raises the distinction I made in the previous chapter concerning the more negative, disabling, failure-inflected connotations of being debilitated vs disabled. I appreciate that this idea moves dangerously close to stigmatising the spectacle of bodies that limp, are blind, cannot walk, and are ageing, but ultimately, this apparent negativity is leading somewhere where the possibility of thinking differently about failure-inflected interpretations beckons. I also want to be true to what I see in Beckett's work by not finding unnecessary silver linings. Of course, a certain degree of the reader's fantasy as the lens of interpretation cannot be avoided, even though I am cautious of interpretations.

Beckett does not attempt to paint a redeeming or uplifting picture of the situation of being impaired or ageing, nor is it one of pity and pathos. It is, however, one of suffering, and in this regard, Beckett's work can be useful in critiquing models of disability that veer away from including suffering and trauma as an experience of impairment. Yet these depictions are not without humanity and relatability, and this is why they resonate so much (for those who find the play resonant). Although *Endgame* has the reputation of being one of the bleakest of Beckett's plays, it is also somewhat comedic, in a disparaging sort of way. Like *Waiting for Godot*, and the physical comedy between Vladimir and Estragon, there is a certain slapstick dimension to the relationship between Hamm and Clov. Clov has a pronounced limp and cannot sit down, which is in contrast to Hamm's inability to stand up. In a darkly comic way, the pair is the perfect match. In this sense, we could say that the physical imperfections complement the characters within a relationality characterised by difference, not the aesthetic of mainstream beauty. As Hamm says, commenting on their respective physical misfortunes, "Every man their speciality" (Beckett, 1958/2006, p. 97). The comedy of physical ailments is a running theme in Beckett's work, where the human subject is not permitted to take up a grandiose position in relation to physicality. Instead, our noses are ground in the dirt, brought into the reality of our imperfections, and not permitted any reprieve. The day-to-day veneer of respectability and the generally hidden boundaries of the body are punctured by references to lice and self-urination. Other ailments are implied through Clov's interactions with Hamm about the state of their mutual physical health:

> Hamm: How are your eyes?
> Clov: Bad.
> Hamm: How are your legs?
> Clov: Bad.
>
> (1958/2006, p. 95)

Hamm is dependent on Clov to help him in his infirmity, and Clov appears emotionally dependent on Hamm, until he makes a move to leave him at the very end of the play, although of course we don't know if he actually leaves. Hamm is not a likeable character, and from the vantage point of his chair, he dominates Clov, ordering him around, blowing his whistle for attendance, and being mean and bad-tempered. He is certainly not a poster boy for disability, as Catanzaro (2007) has observed. Hamm's "high camp version of the paralytic" challenges taboos of representing or denigrating the disabled (p. 175).

The representation of disability within the play is not set within a concrete narrative of why or how this situation occurred. There is no intimation of cause or references to anything being otherwise, although there is a clear indication of suffering and pain; yet, often, in true Beckettian style, it is sarcastically portrayed. It is not clear when Hamm went blind or if he was always so, but somehow, one imagines his physical ailments have been acquired as opposed to congenital. Even the toy dog lacks a leg and cannot stand on the floor. This ubiquitous depiction of infirmity without inferred causation highlights the instability and temporary nature of the able-bodied category, per se. It is a well-known saying in disability studies that everyone is only temporarily able-bodied and that, as a follow-on, we are all universally potentially disabled. As Robert McRuer argues:

> Everyone is virtually disabled, both in the sense that able-bodied norms are "intrinsically impossible to embody" fully and in the sense that able-bodied status is always temporary, disability being the one identity category that all people will embody if they live long enough.
>
> (2006, p. 31)

However, it must be said that being 'virtually disabled', although an ontological potentiality, does not equate with the reality of becoming so. That said, McRuer's statement points to the inevitability of the body failing all of us at some point, in some way, even in the final moments of life. While probably not a deliberate tactic, in not conforming to politically correct representations of disability, Beckett's debilitated bodies challenge some of the emerging narratives of disability that buy into the neoliberal ideal of productivity and achievement. Even within the disability community, there are narratives that deny the fragility or trauma inherent to the body and that speak to an image of the self that transcends obstacles and achieves greatness. In today's times of increasing awareness of equality and disability rights, tropes and recurring images of the ideal disabled person emerge in popular culture. These include narratives of the 'overcomer', the 'Olympian', 'the non-complainer', and the person that, no matter what the disability, is just as 'productive' as everybody else. These images or narrative categories of disabled people are idealised within our culture as hallmarks of how we conceive of value and worth regarding the citizen and the subject. Even disability narratives within discourses (such as the social model of disability) can often deny the reality of physical impairment by working (understandably) to undo the negative associations of such bodies. In contrast, Beckett's bodies are debilitated in such a way as to flaunt an inherently non-productive image of the human, posing a resistance to any conception of an idealised gestalt. This representation could be viewed as both liberating and contemptuous. However, in line with current Beckett scholarship, I would be slow to interpret these bodily manifestations as simply concrete representations or metaphors of disability or indeed figures of disability as metaphors per se. As Siobhan Purcell puts it: "Beckett's and Geulincx's impaired figures are not merely symbols or metaphors for the human condition; they are the *a priori* model of human experience" (2018, pp. 191–192).

Rather than being simply metaphors, the repetition of fragmented and ailing bodies across Beckett's oeuvre is indicative of something symptomatic at the level of representation in relation to a trauma at the level of the body, which poses a question of being. This question of being is refracted through images and tropes that sometimes uphold and sometimes challenge a Cartesian view of the mind-body relation. That the emphasis is more on the body-mind relation, that is, a conception of subjectivity rooted in the somato-psychic perspective, is pertinent to the emphasis Beckett places on the debilitated or disabled body as the backdrop to his characters' outpourings of narrative and memory in so many instances. Whether insight can be gleaned from this relation is another matter, and I do feel that Beckett's characters are sometimes curiously lively in their minds, considering their infirmities. We need to remember, though, that debility and disability cover a multitude of situations and aspects of physical experience. There are situations where a person might be paralysed but be completely agile within their mind and thinking, while in contrast, someone may seem totally mobile but be suffering from extreme cognitive fatigue. Beckett often uses the trope of the fragmented body to question where the self begins or ends. In *The Unnamable,* the narrator describes the experience of confinement without knowledge of the boundary of self: "The sawdust no longer presses against my stumps. I don't know where I end. I left it yesterday" (Beckett, 1953/1978, p. 47).

Interestingly, the same physical image appears in *Endgame,* where Nell and Nagg's visually absent, amputated bodies are situated within the sawdust of their dustbins. The figure of the Beckettian truncated body signifies the human subject as both limited and unlimited, finite and infinite. It is an entity in between life and death. The narrating subject is demarcated by lack, the absence of a body, for example, yet strangely undead, as Beckett's characters go on speaking and thinking despite impossible mind–body scenarios. The contrast between speech or internal narration and the body's position in the environment often disrupts the Cartesian paradigm of rationality or highlights the cogito as potentially farcical. Beckett often takes Descartes' "I think therefore I am" literally, retracting the body as the source of life and cognition, and allowing characters to rave on as part objects or thought automatons. The environments within which these bodies are situated are also pertinent to the aesthetic of debility. Ubersfeld makes the point that Nell and Nagg speaking from the location of a garbage can, for example, serves to undercut the speaker's credibility.

> In Endgame the old men's speeches come out of a garbage can, and the message is less in the speeches than it is in the speech–garbage can relation. What can you say when your message comes out of a garbage can? (1999, p. 162)

Thus, this example implies that the symbolic construction of the stage setting and the juxtaposition of objects and language dislocate habitual associations between form and content. One of these associations is that of time and chronicity.

## Crip Time

The notion of the chronic permeates *Endgame* as a theme of temporality and abjectness. In its state of 'dying on' the body is somewhat of a waste product, a remainder of the slow decomposition of the human being over time. The very fact that we are born introduces us to finite parameters, such as those inherent to the body. The body is a function of time. As an organic entity, our physicality has a finite trajectory and is constantly changing. These changes are largely imperceptible on a day-to-day basis, but ultimately, the trajectory of the body is "taking its course" and subject to the laws of nature. Interestingly, Smith observes that 'old stancher' (what Hamm refers to as his handkerchief) is derived from the word 'stanch', meaning "to stop the flow of blood". From this perspective, the handkerchief becomes a "provisional bandage", an object that signifies the attempt to plug a wound (2007, p. 100). Within this metonymy of associations with suffering, there is also an ambivalence toward time: hope for its quick progression toward an end, but also a desire to slow it down, to resist its erasure.

There is an absence of the anchoring of chronological time in the play; we don't know where or when the events occur, but time is present through the decomposition of forms and the references that Hamm and Clov make to it: "Something is taking its course"; "The time is zero"; "Is it not time for my painkiller?" (Beckett, 1958/2006). Time is what erodes the body, what renders it ultimately powerless to the hands of fate. Ageing and debility are functions of time and speak to the chronicity of any lifespan within the parameters of organic entropy. The bodies in *Endgame* bear the hallmarks of time's chronic progression as little by little, and almost with a divine cynicism, the egoic dreams of immortality and narcissistic mastery are eroded. The juxtaposition of the absence of normative time in the play and the centrality of the debilitated body as a figure of resistance to productivity opens a perspective that Elizabeth Freeman has coined crip temporality. Fundamentally, crip temporality is a version of time inflected by the experiential reality of those living with disabilities, in which time does not always function the same way or at the same pace. As Freeman (2010) argues in her seminal work on queer temporality, *Time Binds*, and then in her later edited collection with Ellen Samuels, *Crip Temporalities* (2021), the notion of temporality is also normative or socially constructed and as subjects of late capitalism, we are subject to the injunctions and dictates placed on our bodies to conform to schedules of time that serve the project of maximum productivity. She coins the term chrononormativity to refer to this normative organisational component of temporality and its materialistic and neoliberal oppressive aim. Crip temporality, on the other hand, refers to a version of time that takes account of difference, slowness, ways of doing things that do not conform to the standard able-bodied conception of productivity. Furthermore, it is worth noting that, as Freeman argues in *Theorising the Chronic*,[2] including its temporal resonances, the word chronic is also indicative of certain intransigent bodily states such as illness, disease and debility, deficits of character and ill-fated occurrences (2011, p. 3). Freeman makes an argument for recognising the labour involved in enduring such states over time and, by so doing, counteracts stigmatised notions of the disabled body as being unproductive, lazy, or malingering. In other words, for many people, the state of illness/disability and its daily challenges of survival, including often enduring physical pain and debility, is a form of labour and work in itself. Just being, in and of itself, without any additional physical challenges, can be a form of labour, where living involves an expenditure of effort to manage the energy of the general internal clamour of the drives as they seek satisfaction around the continual and necessary non-rapport of encountering the absent object of desire. In fact, work in a normative sense is generally an escape from the existential labour of being, the enduring of the dissatisfactions of the body and the impossible satisfactions of the drives. While it may be a stretch of the imagination to say that Beckett exhibits debilitated bodies as a form of a crip aesthetic to illustrate the very labour of being, as a 'being there' through the suffering of the body, it is certainly tempting to impose a notion of crip time onto the chronotopic planes of embodiment situated within his drama. That the time is zero in *Endgame* and that the bodies of the characters are reduced to ground zero certainly lends credence to the possible operation of an alternate form of time, one that does not conform to the historico-logical linear trajectory of conventional time. This dimension of time may be more embodied, slowed down by immobility or the ruptures of pain and functional challenges, subject to the recursions of memory, the retroactive epiphanies of recall, and the a-temporality of the unconscious. Crip time can also be time accelerated, as Margaret Price (2015) argues in her elaborations of the body–mind problem. Within *Endgame* however, this is not a presentation of time with endless possibility and a naïve optimism of queer alternality but rather a vision of humanity that suffers *from* time, from the inherent choices attendant to the state of being, the need to act, even when all acts are futile and finite, 'there is no more'. The fact that the characters are suffering existentially (from waiting, time, and being) as well as directly from the body (pain, infirmity, ill health) is evident in their wish to end it all and in the misery referred to directly by Hamm and Clov.

> Clov: He's crying.
> Hamm: Then he's living.
> Hamm: Did you ever have an instant of happiness?...
> Clov: Not to my knowledge.
>
> (Beckett, 1958/2006, p. 123)

That Hamm and Clov are suffering is evident, as is their desire to bring an end to this suffering, and yet they can't:

> Hamm: Why don't you kill me?
> Clov: I don't know the combination of the larder.
>
> (Beckett, 1958/2006, p. 110)

Beckett's sardonic humour about wanting to end but not being able to allows us to approach the realisation that, as White states, "To be physical is to suffer, and Beckett illustrates the pain of existence, denying us the possibility that death may provide a release" (2009, p. 3). White also makes the curious and somewhat darkly optimistic point that the physical ailments of the characters of *Endgame* are a source of hope, as they are portents for the drawing near of death and the possible soon release from the enclosure of the body. This of course raises the question of the representation of disability being associated with death, and the figures of debility, falling into the ableist-normative medicalising narrative, where disability is a disease, a defect, a failing of sorts. I'm aware my own reading could be categorised that way, and I do, admittedly, associate suffering and trauma with debility and disability. However, as I have been arguing, failure, as it relates to the body, does not have to be considered as inherently negative in a moralistic sense or something that is the opposite of success but rather points to a gap, a chasm at the heart of the symbolic, an encounter with the Real. There is failure beneath our speech, literally, as we grapple for words to describe the lack of an object we can never recover, no matter what we strive to achieve. We should reconsider negativity and failure as ontological givens, as their exposure often points to the heart of our existence. And yet it is in the negativity or hopelessness of the atmosphere of *Endgame* that something of being is rendered visible. What happens when all our distractions run aground, when all our painkillers, either as palliations for physical pain or the habits that accompany quotidian existence, run out, and we are left with ourselves, the body, our infirmities?

## The Pain of Existing

Despite its comic allusions, *Endgame* depicts a scene of desolation, an erasure of the old world order, the ending of possibilities, a site of futile action and a morbid vision of humanity. While it might sound trite to say that desolation has its upside, the subtraction of forms that *Endgame* enacts paves a path to considering how negation, the collapse of the supports of the imaginary dimension of subjectivity, one of which is the world as an entity, engenders an encounter with the rawness of the self, what Lacan has referred to in *Seminar VI*, the seminar on desire as the "pain of existing" or existing when desire is no longer present (Lacan, Lesson 5, 10 December 1958–1959, p. 63). While the characters in *Endgame* may not be said to be on the level of mourning indicative of the state Lacan is describing through the example of Hamlet in *Seminar VI*, that is, I'm not sure we really say that fantasy has collapsed for the characters and they are confronting the core of their being, the play nonetheless depicts a scenario where this may occur. Certainly the structures that support a world and being are collapsing or closing in through the slow encroachment of loss, absence and catastrophic resonances. We could say that *Endgame* stages the conditions of possibility for a collapse in the coordinates of subjective fantasy without being this collapse. This is where it gives grounds for hope. In *Endgame*, existence is almost reduced to the body; there is very little to desire, apart from the end itself, and through the loss of all that may give pleasure, desire may run aground, leaving the subject at the mercy of the drives. Desire is in some way a defence against the drive. While in *Seminar VI*, Lacan names the pain of existing, in the seminar on ethics, *Seminar VII*, desolation is pivoted within an ethical frame, where the end of analysis is described by Lacan as a form of intense anguish, or subjective destitution.[3] The pain of existing is pertinent for all subjects; it is, in some sense, the bedrock of being. At any time, for any subject, it can be triggered by intense grief, the loss of a particular person, or, indeed, the loss of physical ability, the impact of an event at the level of the body. According to this perspective, pain is what underlies our existence; it emerges when the fantasy surrounding the big Other collapses, when the object a is no longer the veiled object that sustains desire but is revealed as the painful presence of lack that it really is. Does this mean that *Endgame* illustrates a scenario like the end of analysis? Not specifically, as it is still in the realm of the imaginary, and we are not dealing with an analytical situation to state the obvious. However, I think that in Beckett's work in general, but also in this particular case of *Endgame*, the aesthetic of debility is a phantasmatical attempt to expose this lack beneath fantasy, the loss that subtends the imaginary pillars of identification, the vulnerability of the subject to the drives, the pain of existing that is the affect of being. I say it is phantasmatic as the visual dimension of theatre works to provide the spectator and the author with an object of desire, the spectacle itself, so the vision presented can never actually be devoid of fantasy (the orientation that subtends desire), but this is where this theory becomes paradoxical: given the Real is beyond representation, something of that Real can still be accessed or a recognition induced through the imaginary and symbolic axes of theatre. In some respects, Beckett comes as close as is possible to exposing the Real through the imaginary. For example, thinking of the debilitated bodies in *Endgame*, something of what we repress regarding the vulnerability of the body to ageing, disease, ill health is writ large in such a way that we are not provided with any means to escape this reality. Neither, for that matter, are Hamm and Clov, Nell and Nag. Not even a narrative of heroic overcoming can provide relief in this environment. The absence of Hamm's painkiller is very symbolic in this context of debility as it signifies that which could bring temporary relief to a physical form of suffering or pain while being symbolic of other levels of pain, such as emotional, mental, or simply existential. This basic lack of pain relief can symbolise the absence of distraction from the void, from the jouissance of the body, to which the characters are more at the mercy due to their hemmed-in condition.

Critics such as Russell Smith have commented on the themes of loss, mourning and melancholia within the play. Smith conjectures that *Endgame* portrays the aftermath of a historical catastrophe, with a few remaining survivors left in its wake. While *Endgame* is certainly a play that features loss, the loss of everyday objects to support existence, the loss of physical ability and the destruction of the world as a habitable environment, I view this theme of loss as situated more ontologically than historically. Although no subject exists in a historical vacuum, the same is true of the modality or style of theatre and the nature of viewing reception. In other words, we are dealing with a loss at the level of the body and the subject's relation to language and satisfaction. In this eradication of phenomena, the almost sensory deprivation of the characters, the minimalistic setting, traces out the contours of an absence, represented by the repeated phrase "there's no more." Rather, in viewing loss as something subjective, atemporal or psychical, the repetition of this phrase as it relates to objects signifies the futility of substitution in ever reaching a satisfaction of desire or even of providing an illusion of satisfaction. For that is the function of objects of desire. There can be no ultimate satisfaction, as desire is always metonymical, moving from one object to another. This metonymy is laid bare in *Endgame*, as one by one objects are presented and then rejected as not being present, as non-existent. There are no more objects that can punctuate and palliate the eroding progression of time; the body is laid bare in its suffering of the drives. What I am implying here through the situation of the play is that in states of debilitation and disability, we may be more prone to the angst of the drives as they clamour for satisfaction.[4] In *Endgame*, as in many plays, Beckett manages to carve out the place of symbolic absence through the materiality of forms and corresponding linguistic devices. The very conditions of meaning are laid bare in order to be eroded, leaving both an absence as a figurative loss and yet a space for possibility. This space for possibility is borne of an encounter with desolation, an encounter we could say is ethical in a Lacanian sense if, through this eradication of forms and the content of the sensory world, it lays bare our desire or allows us to glimpse it even for a moment. We remember that for Lacan, the unconscious operates in flashes and ruptures, disruptions and mistakes, with the subject of the unconscious making its presence felt not as a positive entity but as that which opposes conscious thought. So is there an ethical dimension to *Endgame*? Is it within the very structure of the play itself, or is it a function of the dialectic between the play and the spectator? This seemingly perplexing question of a play that resists interpretation and its ethical import has been posed by other critics. Ben Ware has observed (2015):

> We might ask, following Theodor Adorno (1991, 244): how is it possible to ascertain ethical significance in a work in which "humankind continues to vegetate, creeping along after events that even the survivors cannot really survive, on a rubbish heap that has made even reflection on one's own damaged state useless"?
>
> (p. 3)

I think it is in the very profundity of the palimpsest-like series of losses, from which there is very little relief, in which the survivors are struggling to survive, that the ethical import is found. How to go on living when all is almost lost? To be clear, it is not so much the representation of disabled or debilitated bodies that is ethical, as I think this has been proven to be questionable by Beckett scholars—*Endgame* is "not a play that a disabled person wants to see, if they want to see something positive about themselves (interview, 2017,

Chapter Two)" (quoted in Simpson, p. 209). However, in my view, the ethical dimension is in the staging of an encounter with nothingness, a nothingness that is also encapsulated by the body as it tends towards ground zero. In this 'corpsed' environment, in which Hamm and Clov are situated, we encounter a scenario of ultimate dread, where Hamm and Clov express the frustration of an experience that never seems to end, similar to Vladimir and Estragon in *Waiting for Godot*. Indeed, while there are other similarities between the plays, such as a quasi pseudo-couple who abuse each other to pass the time and the uncertainty of what is to come, *Endgame* moves further along the axis of nothingness, where not even the promise of Godot awaits. This staging of coming and going, or rather coming and *not* going, is characteristic of Beckett's work, the dialectics of which create a discontinuity of relations, a drama of missed encounters. It is important to stress that the ethical dimension of *Endgame* is not necessarily experienced as a 'happy outcome' of watching a play; nonetheless, I think that there is room for a certain loosening of illusion on the part of the spectator, not least as it concerns the pervasive expectation of seeing able bodies performing. While I feel there is something ethical in this portrayal of devastation and that possibility lurks within the crevices of despair, I would not want to make assumptions or draw simplistic conclusions that all representations of failure comprise some sort of enlightening epiphany that could be used for activist means or as a liberation from stigma, for example. As Thomas Mansell says in his essay on *Endgame*, "Beckett's writing is frequently indifferent, often callously so, to people's more obvious hardships, devoting excessive attention instead to coincidental features of their situation" (2007, p. 12). While this is harsh criticism and I think Beckett also displays great humanity in presenting these scenarios of hardship, as I think his own self-reflection is intrinsic to these seeming admonishments, it should be borne in mind to offset utopic notions surrounding the presence of the disabled body in the Beckettian terrain. Tendencies to utopic thinking can also be a response to the pain of existing, as remaining without meaning is difficult. While I have been discussing pain here in a more existential sense, in the next chapter on Artaud, pain takes on a more affective dimension as a modality of theatrical performance and pathway of the body's relation to being.

## Notes

1 We should note that the stage directions place Hamm in a chair with castors, not a wheelchair. Hannah Simpson (2022) makes the point, and I have also noticed, how frequently critics misread this chair as a wheelchair. Although Hamm does at one point say that he would like a real wheelchair, Simpson argues that this misreading underlines the salient place of disability in the play. It also suggests a very particular association with immobility and of aligning disability with wheelchairs. As if the wheelchair is the sine qua non of disability. Not everyone with limited mobility or who may be debilitated uses a wheelchair.

2 This reference was a talk given by the late Elizabeth Freeman at UCD (University College Dublin) and the paper was sent through personal correspondence.

3 Verhaeghe & Declercq (2002) make the point that subjective destitution was never elaborated by Lacan and is well-know more as the result of Slavoj Žižek's extensive commentaries on it.

4 This presupposes two questions: what do I mean by drive/s and why would a person be more subject to them in states of debilitation? We saw in chapter 3 that the concept of the drive derives from Freud's first conceptualisations of it as something on the border of the psyche and the soma, a force that causes a demand placed on the mind/psyche for work. As an endogenous excitation, the drive can be experienced as discomfort/pain, trauma even, as the libidinal energy associated with it seeks release. I mentioned earlier that in states of illness, the ego may suffer fatigue or innervation in some way, leading to increased potential for melancholy, depression or anxiety. Perhaps apart from the loss associated with illness/disability, there is the potential for increased drive activity as a consequence of a reduction of release mechanisms, for example, through exercise or other activities where drive impulses may be channelled. Of course, there is also the case that a person experiencing debility, pain, illness or disability has an increased pain threshold due to their condition and may have an increased capacity to manage jouissance.

## References


Beckett, S. (1958). *Endgame*. Grove Press.

Beckett, S. (1953/2006). Waiting for Godot. In *Samuel Beckett. The complete dramatic works* (pp. 7–89). Faber & Faber.

Beckett, S. (1953/1978). *The unnamable*. Grove Press.

Catanzaro, F. M. (2007). Masking and the social construct of the body in Samuel Beckett's Endgame. In M. Byron (Ed.), *Samuel Beckett's Endgame* (pp. 165–189). New York: Rodopi.

Freeman, E. (2011). *Theorising the Chronic*: Unpublished.

Kumar, K. J. (1997). The chess metaphor in Samuel Beckett's endgame. *Modern Drama*, 40 (4), 540–552.

Kristeva, J. (1982). *Powers of horror: An essay on abjection* (I.S. Rouidiez, Transl.). New York: Columbia University Press.

Lacan, J. (1958–1959). *The seminar of Jacques Lacan. Book VI: Desire and its interpretation*. Transl. C. Gallagher. Unpublished.

Mansell, T. (2007). Hard-to-hear music in Endgame. In M.S. Byron (Ed.) *Samuel Beckett's Endgame*. Rodopi.

McRuer, R (2006). *Crip theory: Cultural signs of queerness and disability*. New York and London: New York University Press.

Price, M. (2015).The bodymind problem and the possibilities of pain. *Hypatia* 30,(1), 268–284.

Purcell, S. (2018). *"Extraordinary debilities": Disability in the works of Samuel Beckett*. Unpublished PhD Thesis NUIG: Galway.

Simpson, H. (2022). *Samuel Beckett and disability performance*. Palgrave Macmillan

Smith, R. (2007). Endgame's remainders. In M.S. Byron (Ed.), *Samuel Beckett's Endgame*. (pp. 99–101). New York: Rodopi.

Ubersfeld, A. (1999). *Reading theatre*. (F. Collins, Trans.) Toronto: University of Toronto Press.

Verhaeghe, P. & Declercq, F. (2002). Lacan's analytical goal: "Le Sinthome" or the feminine way. In: L. Thurston (ed.), *Essays on the final Lacan. Re-inventing the symptom.* New York: The Other Press, pp. 59–83.
Ware, B. (2015). Tragic-dialectical-perfectionism: on the ethics of Beckett's *Endgame. College Literature*, 42 (1), 3–22.
White, K. (2009). *Beckett and decay.* Continuum International Literary Studies.

Chapter 6

# Artaud's Impossible Body

## Cruelty, Pain, and Affect

While the body is a universal trauma for all human beings, it is usually covered by a veil of fantasy. For the writer and playwright Antonin Artaud, this veil is removed, and the body emerges as a source of pain, suffering, and transcendence, both as a lived reality and as an ideal within his theatrical aesthetic. The finale of Beckett's *Endgame*, which reveals the pain of existing as a state of being conceived when all external phenomena are pared away, is a fitting segue into the work of Artaud, for whom pain, both physical and mental, is a critical signifier. However, the pain of existing is situated differently within Artaud's aesthetic compared to Beckett's, and this difference sheds light on particular orientations vis-à-vis the body or the body–mind connection in their work. For Beckett, the aesthetic of debility/disability acts as a form of negation, a trope of failure or something not working out in the Real, through which a path towards the negativity of being is forged. For Artaud, a pathway to considering being is also opened out through the body; his theatrical aesthetic is one in which the body is centre stage as the medium through which he wished to transcend the limiting, rationalising, psychologising modality of language in the Western theatre. Rather than figuring absence and the negativity of being, it is one of excess, where being is aligned with the seeming substance of the body. His writings on theatre demonstrate his conflictual relation to thought, as something representative, and to materiality, as that which relates to the substance of the organism. Through his theory of a Theatre of Cruelty, we can trace the impetus towards the invention of an impossible body, a body that speaks in the language of affects and signs, signals and hieroglyphs. Affect, pain, and jouissance combine in Artaud's work to create an aesthetic of excess that reveals the drive to reduce the discordance between the subject and the body. Through Artaud's metaphysical quest, the role of affect as a signifier of bodily truth is situated within a mind–body narrative that elevates the body to a conduit of hidden meanings. In this sense, the body becomes a solution to the enigma of being.

DOI: 10.4324/9781003509622-9

## Between Thought and Being

One of the distinguishing factors of Artaud's bodily aesthetics is how he places himself or his own suffering at the centre of his writings and artistic works. Whether Artaud's body of writings, letters, and plays can be called artistic work or at times a symptom of mental distress has been addressed by Ros Murray (2014), particularly in consideration of the spells he produced through psychosis, but certainly his writings have a deeply personal quality and most likely served as a stabilising function in his life or at least may have kept him alive. Although deeply ambivalent about writing and language, "all writing is garbage" (Artaud, p. 85), it is through writing that Artaud manages to frame the inexpressible and through words that he conveys an image of the body that transcends human form. As Murray also points out, Artaud's work attempts to materialise something of inner experience, to place the body into writing as corporeal traces, sounds and utterances that give voice to bodily processes. There is a tension here, I think, in that Artaud was attempting to ground himself and locate thought, that which escaped him in words, in the material, corporeal substance of the body, while also acknowledging and refusing the body as a source of suffering. In his earlier work and letters to Jacques Rivière, Artaud speaks of his struggle to anchor his thought in being:

> But thinking means something more to me than not being completely dead. It means being in touch with oneself at every moment; it means not ceasing for a single moment to feel oneself in one's inmost being, in the unformulated mass of one's life, in the substance of one's reality; it means not feeling in oneself an enormous hole, a crucial absence; it means always feeling one's thought equal to one's thought, however inadequate the form one is able to give it. But my thinking sins not only because of its weakness, but also because of its quantity. I always think at an inferior rate.
>
> (Artaud, 1976, p. 70)

We can note here that Artaud refers to an attempt to align thought and feeling, and crucially, the desire not to feel an enormous hole in being through a certain identification of thought with itself. There is often remarkable insight and expressive perspicacity within Artaud's writings that challenge the conception of him as a madman. Of course, being mad and insightful need not be mutually exclusive, but they are often not seen as co-existing. The desire to cover the hole in being is clear from Artaud's words: he wants to align thought with the innermost being; however, this may be an impossible quest. As I have already shown through Lacanian thinking, being does not align with thought. As Lacan puts it:

> Being cannot be grasped as thought except in an alternating fashion. It is in a succession of alternating moments that he thinks, that his memory

> appropriates its thinking reality without this thinking being at any moment able to join up with itself in its own certainty.
>
> (Lacan, Lesson 2, 22 November 1961–62), p. 16

However, the fact that this may be a universal truth of the human condition does not diminish its acuteness for Artaud or the urgency with which a disturbance at the level of the ego or thought may have impacted him. This disturbance was expressed through an ambiguous relation to the body as both relief for and agent of suffering, which can be illustrated by the fact that he was an opium addict for most of his life—a scenario of pleasure and pain at the level of the organism. This is something I think should be emphasised when understanding his relation to the body within his writings and the drive behind the Theatre of Cruelty. This ambivalent position of the body in addiction can provide insight into his aesthetic of cruelty—a cruelty that contains a drive to jouissance—a vision that has captivated the imaginations of so many. In brief, jouissance is that beyond to the pleasure principle, an enjoyment in suffering or a too muchness that renders the subject at the mercy of repetition and symptomatic release. The drive to jouissance features heavily in Artaud's life and aesthetics. Although a notoriously difficult concept to tie down and, as Leader (2021) argues, often a shorthand for obfuscating the complexity of pain, suffering, and pleasure, I will briefly refer here to a distinction of jouissances. The body or the organism is a source of intrinsic jouissance, what I would call the existential jouissance of the flesh, but through drug-taking, it can also be manipulated to produce an intoxicated jouissance, pleasure/satisfaction of an intensity that has an almost morbid quality to it. While I cannot go into a detailed analysis of the role of addiction in Artaud's life, I think it is relevant to bear it in mind as another avenue where he tried to reinvent, intervene, or go beyond the confines of the organic body.[1] It might sound strange to use the word reinvent in relation to drug-taking, but in essence, often people are trying to become someone else, or anesthetise the preexisting self to create an altered persona or sense of being. We could even say that there is a form of creativity involved as well as destruction. In other words, through his work and the various artistic mediums he engaged with, he attempts to invent a new body from the destruction of the body formulated by language through the lack-inducing structure of the symbolic order. This project of reinventing the body begins with his articulations of pain and suffering, takes form in his invention of a corporeal theatre and is specularised in his famous phrase "the body without organs", which features in his 1947 radio work *To Have Done with the Judgement of God*. In a later chapter, I will concentrate more specifically on the idea of the reinvention of a new body through the body without organs as it arises in this performance, but for the moment, it is important to contextualise Artaud's theatrical work as a corporeal project of transcendence, and to examine its captivating appeal and inherent failure. The Theatre of Cruelty was not simply an art form but a mode of being—a way to exist with the body. As Susan Sontag points out, for Artaud, theatre was a means of healing "the split between language and flesh" (1976, xxxv). Ironically this was to be achieved through the concept of cruelty.

## Cruelty: A Theatre of Excess

Despite his copious writings and poetry, for certain audiences, Artaud is most famous for his vision or manifesto for theatre, the Theatre of Cruelty, rather than its implementation as a staged phenomenon. Artaud's invention of a theatre that could "assault the senses" and act on the nerves of the spectator really only comes to fruition in one staged play, *The Cenci,* which I will discuss in detail in the next chapter and which, from an audience perspective, has been judged to be a failure. While his earlier plays, like *Le Jet du Sang* [The Spurt of Blood] (1925), contain resonances of the manifesto for cruelty, it was never staged in his lifetime. That Artaud's theatrical vision may be unstageable is an intriguing fact, and it begs the question of what it is about this vision and the signifier of cruelty that so captivates a theatrical and academic audience. What may spring to mind when we hear the word 'cruelty' is the harm caused by one person to another; it is not simply about a state of pain or suffering, but about suffering inflicted on one person by another in an abusive and excessive way. Yet, according to Artaud, the cruelty he refers to is first directed at himself and is not violent in a physical sense; rather, it reveals to the audience the harsh contingencies of life. In his essay, "The Theatre of Cruelty" (First Manifesto), Artaud is clear about this. It is worth quoting in full:

> This is why I propose a theatre of cruelty. With that mania for depreciating everything that we all have today, as soon as I uttered the word 'cruelty' everyone immediately took it to mean 'blood'. But 'theatre of cruelty' means a theatre that is difficult and cruel first of all for myself. And on the level of representation it is not a question of that cruelty which we can practice on each other by cutting up each other's bodies, by sawing away at our personal anatomies, or, like Assyrian emperors, by sending each other packages of human ears, noses, or neatly severed nostrils through the mail, but of that much more terrible and necessary cruelty which things can practice on us. We are not free. And the sky can still fall on our heads. And the theatre has been created to teach us, first of all, that.
>
> (Artaud, 1976/1932, p. 256)

So, cruelty here relates to a somewhat deterministic worldview from which we are not free and cannot escape, rather than physical torture or specific bodily harm. Artaud clearly wanted the theatre to awaken the spectator to the reality of the sufferings of life, a life in which we are subject to chance and unfortunate contingencies, without providing rational explanations or neatly formulated plots that mitigate the shock of the cruelty of life. One of the critical distinctions to note regarding Artaud's theatre and its historical place within performance studies is the role of the spectacle in the dialectic between art form and spectator. Artaud wanted to bridge the gap between art and life, where theatre could have, in his words, an almost magical quality, performed through force, something more than representation. The Theatre of Cruelty invoked the spectacle as the affective means of impacting the spectator beyond the distance generated by language, unlike what Aristotle proposed in the *Poetics* as the making of a good tragedy, which did not involve the spectacle:

> It is possible for the evocation of fear and pity to result from the spectacle, and also from the structure of the event itself. The latter is preferable and is the mark of a better poet[…] Those who use spectacle to produce an effect which is not evocative of fear, but simply monstrous, have nothing to do with tragedy; one should not seek every pleasure from tragedy, but the one that is characteristic of it.
>
> (Aristotle, c.335 BC/1996, p. 22)

For Aristotle, the production of a good tragedy involved order, stipulating rules and guidelines for theatre to provoke catharsis. For fear of being reductive about one of the most ambiguous concepts in theatrical discourse, catharsis, in Aristotelian terms, connotes an emotional release brought about by the provocation of the emotions of pity and fear within the context of tragedy. As Maria Grazia Turri (2015) explains, the debate around catharsis has concerned whether Aristotle meant perfection of emotion within the mind or as an abreaction of the mind. Its etymological meaning is 'to purge', as in a medical context, and Turri juxtaposes the concept in psychoanalytic terms, drawing associations with transference and the abreaction of past events in analysis. What is relevant here is that, in contrast to the Aristotelian model of catharsis, Artaud emphatically uses the theatrical spectacle as a means to provoke bodily effects in the audience and to communicate in a universal language of corporeal signs. This is not a catharsis of the mind, where the spectator could take distance from events through pity and fear but an overwhelming of the senses, a shocking encounter designed to rouse the spectator from the inertia of Occidental ennui. We could call Artaud's intent a jouissance of the spectacle, an intense effect/affect that theoretically takes the spectator beyond the pleasure principle aligned with a view of reception as entertainment, where pleasure is a reduction of tension and jouissance is an enjoyment within an excess of tension. Whereas Aristotle was concerned with matters of harmony and moderation, there is an appeal to disorder in Artaud's theatrics that exalts in an excess of the theatrical principle.

Instead of holding the 'mirror up to nature' and conjuring a theatrical copy of reality, Artaud wanted the stage to be part of nature, a double of life, not just a reflection. As Morfee puts it, "All Artaud's writing is profoundly influenced by the idea of replacing representation with performance" (2005, p. 5). The medium of performance, as Artaud points out, allows for actions to occur only once, to avoid the repetition induced by written language and to conjure an originality that theoretically could avoid the stain of the Other's desire as the shadow cast upon the signifiers that subtend the symbolic. We could say that through performance, both within theatre and as a feature of his writings, Artaud wanted to invent a new symbolic order, one where the distance or the sliding between signifier and signified was mediated by a knowledge inscribed on the body, where thought, as that seeming component of the rational dimension of the self, was subverted to the materiality of a language that communicated directly.

> It has not been definitively proved that the language of words is the best possible language. And it seems that on the stage, which is above all a space to fill and a place where something happens, the language of words may have to give way before a language of signs whose objective aspect is the one that has the most immediate impact upon us.
>
> (Artaud, 1938/1958, p. 107)

In this passage, Artaud describes how theatrical performance provides a means of cultivating a new language, one that is composed of signs rather than words. What does this mean exactly? We need to consider the difference between a word/signifier and a sign. In Saussurian terms, a signifier is the vocal sound image of a concept and a sign is that which combines the signifier and the signified—it has a fixed meaning. Artaud states that these signs will have an immediate impact on us, unlike the more rational/psychologising aspect of thought, which words represent. Artaud frequently writes of the dissonances within his thought process, as if he were unable to fully capture and express them in words. There is also a split between the word and the thing, or the thought and the signifier. Instead of this split being symbolised in language, as imperfect representations are, he wanted to embody it, externalise it, and potentially contain or anchor this fragmented part of the self. It seems that in attempting to invent a universal language that could communicate somewhere between gesture and thought, Artaud believed in meaning, albeit conveyed in incandescent ways. Through the medium of performance, he wanted to create a signifying system composed of gestures and bodily signs, affects and the intensity of experience, in which something of the body could be both represented and transcended. Artaud's gestural language of performance, his "syntax of bodily drives" (Morfee p. 5), extends the signification of the physical body beyond the semantical impositions of everyday linguistic sense. In attempting to move beyond words, Artaud placed emphasis on gesture and physical movement as an alternative modality of representation to language. Having been greatly influenced by the Balinese and Oriental style of performance, he incorporated these bodily movements of dance and gesture into a repertoire of physical theatre. However, as Elam argues, gesture and language are not separate but complementary semiotic agents within theatrical discourse:

> Despite Artaud's insistence on an absolute semiotic polarity between language and gesture in the theatre, the fact remains that, except in extreme cases of gestural autonomy (mime), the two are bound to cooperate in the production of theatrical discourse.
>
> (2005, p. 45)

Therefore, although language serves to delimit the perimeters of what can be said, the realm of signification as related to the structure of language may not have been as narrow as Artaud envisaged. A signifier is something that can encompass more than words; it can also be, as Chiesa (2007) puts it, a gesture, a sound, or a bodily movement. "Human body language—for example, shaking one's head, nodding, waving, and so on—insofar as it is equivocal, can also work as a signifier" (p. 50). From this perspective, language is not reduced to actual words or sounds but is a signification system that already extends beyond words. Consequently, Artaud's distinction between body movement/gestures and the psychological and mental properties of words becomes tenuous.

The excessive quality of Artaud's dramaturgy is comparable to the style of his drawings and paintings in his later period, in which the available space on the paper is filled to the utmost. The cramming of space with objects metaphorically diminishes the room that might be left for absence or gaps, illustrating the difficulty of confronting a hole, which, I contend, was endemic to his relationship with language. He states it clearly in *Theatre and Its Double*:

> And just as there will be no unoccupied point in space, there will be neither respite nor vacancy in the spectator's mind or sensibility. That is, between life and the theatre there will be no distinct division, but instead a continuity.
>
> (1938/1958, p. 126)

Artaud's desire for continuity between life and theatre is exemplified by his instruction that the theatre space should extend into the audience and "physically envelop the spectator and immerse them in a constant bath of light, images, movements, and noises" (1938/1958, p. 126). This type of continuity between performance and the spectator attempted to break down the distinction between subject and object and ultimately between life and art. The 'organs' of the Theatre of Cruelty should infiltrate the body, as in the contagion of a plague, extending it beyond the limits of everyday reality, where theatre is more real than life itself.

In his conception of cruelty, Artaud wanted to assault the spectator with the double of life on stage, a spectacle so intense it could potentially liberate the viewer and himself from unconscious conflicts.[2] This was a style of theatre that would shock people through the body, shaking them up from the habitual inertia of the everyday; a metaphysical project of transcendence:

> To make metaphysics out of a spoken language is to make the language express what it does not ordinarily express: to make use of it in a new, exceptional, and unaccustomed fashion; to reveal its possibilities for producing physical shock.
>
> (Artaud, 1938/1958, p. 46)

This quote reveals a certain ambiguity concerning language for Artaud. It is not completely without the capacity to communicate or express certain realities but it must be employed in such a way as to produce an effect on the body. What could this physical shock be but something in the realm of affect—that is, feeling with associated bodily sensations—or vice versa?

## Affect and the Gap in Being

In his writings, Artaud shows a preoccupation with the body's physical processes and waste products, with "caca" a regular feature. Furthermore, these physical processes are associated with being: "There where it smells of shit, it smells of being" (Artaud, 1947/1976, p. 559). Artaud regularly attributes a physical and abject materiality to being—it has the resonance of a substance, something tangible. The physical processes of the body appear to ground Artaud in being and by so doing circumvent or re-suture the split between representation (thought) and the physical body. In essence, he wanted to bring thought to the level of physical processes, the nerves that subtend all life, to overturn rationality through the passions of the flesh. A philosophical question arises: is Artaud's work Cartesian, presupposing a divide between body and mind, or is it a means of addressing the split engendered by the cogito concerning rationality vs feeling? Descartes did not simply posit the rational thinking subject as separate from the body but also fundamentally left affect or feeling out of the equation—the 'I' was not a feeling subject. According to Antonio Damasio (1994) in *Descartes' Error*, in which he argues for the neurophysiological integration of feeling and rationality, we cannot have rationality without feeling. Damage to parts of the brain that control feelings can affect our ability to make cognitive decisions. This is relevant when considering how Artaud seeks to transcend rationality through a language of corporeal signs and hieroglyphs, one that cannot be reduced to mental constructs. In short, Artaud's metaphysical project is both a response to the Cartesian influence on Western thought and the division between mind and body but manages to overshoot it and, instead of undoing the split between mind and body, reinforces it by imagining that rationality and the organic body are separate rather than already intrinsically connected. In essence, Artaud's error may be to idealise the organic body as a source of truth, a means by which thought, as a secondary process, could be reconciled with matter as immanence. So in other words, he attempts to ground the Real of the body, that which is outside of language, within being, which is also a function of language. There is a further complication in thinking through the Cartesian resonances or critique within Artaud's writings. We saw in Chapter 3 that there is a Cartesian element to psychoanalytic thinking regarding the discord between the unconscious/the subject, on the one hand, and the body, on the other. It's not that there is a split between mind and body, but that we are dealing with a polyvalence of variables that operate on different registers simultaneously. We only have to think of Lacan's Borromean knot and how the Real, the Imaginary and the Symbolic overlap in a topological rather than linear way to consider the atemporality or simultaneity of subjectivity. The divided subject is split between the conscious and the unconscious, but I argue that this has implications for conceptualising being, and that, in effect, being is not a unitary concept but is bifurcated—the being of the body and the being of the subject. The unconscious mediates these two modalities of being. Also, it creates a sense of division or noncoincidence between subject and body. The subject, born of the discourse of the Other, cannot be reduced to the organic body, although it is inscribed on it. While the subject is a lack of being, induced by the trauma of the signifier, in my view, the being of the organic body is pure jouissance before the letter. Just as affect is aligned with consciousness in Mark Solms' neuropsychoanalytic view, I argue jouissance is a felt sense, the background condition of the life force. This split between the being of the subject and that of the body is represented, in Lacanian terms, by the concept of the object a as that which forms the matheme of the fantasy, with the divided subject positioned in relation to a desire that masks the lack in being. The object a is the remainder of a body, the fallout from the castrating function of language that creates a body subject to the laws and borders of the symbolic. In essence, I think that Artaud attempts to bypass the symbolic loss of this object through an enjoyment at the level of the organism, in the form of shit/caca, pain/suffering and general excessive sensation. To put it simply, what do people do when their very being as subjects is in question? When thought appears disjunct from the self, disordered and destabilised and a sense of unreality or free-floating in an amorphous consciousness prevails. Often it is the sensations of the organic body that are brought to bear to establish an anchor in the world. To feel pain or suffering at a physical level can induce a sense of concrete reality, an immediacy of attention, a distraction from the realm of thought. These lost objects of the body are effectively materialised to plug the gap in being engendered by language. This 'suturing' through performance is attempted through the invocation of affect and bodily excess as transmitters of an altered state. Whereas Beckett frames the empty space of the subject's being through the staged characteristics of minimalism, absence, and silence, Artaud attempts to fill the silence, blocking out all lack. What may make this analysis complex and hard to follow is that the body, as we have seen in Lacanian terms, is composed of signifiers, imaginary identifications and a Real or enjoying jouissance substance. Therefore what does it mean to speak of the presence or absence of the body in these terms? As the object a (that object in the Real) bears a fundamental relationship to the body through its derivation of drive objects, such as the voice, gaze, and shit, the presence or absence of the body transcends the limits of material corporeality. It is to be found in the derivations of the body, which can be dislocated from materiality. I argue that a play itself can contain an orientation in relation to the object a and the Other of language, and that the body is not just read as an organic entity on the stage but as something that leaves traces and residues within the dramatic structure. In other words, we can identify the relation to the object a in the deformations of the imaginary engendered by the theatrical performance. For example, the explosive sounds in Artaud's theatre are designed to bypass the limitations of language and instead cultivate an affect in the body, as a means of short-circuiting the lack inherent to words and linguistic signifiers. Artaud's language conveys an overwhelming of the body of the spectator:

> I propose then a theatre in which violent physical images crush and hypnotise the sensibility of the spectator, seized by the theatre as by a whirlwind of higher forces.
>
> (Artaud, 1938/1958, p. 83)

In Artaud's dramatic vision, the spectacle of performance is idealised as a vehicle through which the being of the body can be accessed in its immediacy. Immediacy and non-repetition are very much a feature of the performative gesture. In his ambition for an "affective athleticism" (1938/1958, p.133), theatre may bypass the stagnation of static images and forms. As Artaud states: "This means that in the theatre more than anywhere else it is the affective world of which the actor must be aware, ascribing to it virtues which are not those of an image but carry a material sense" (1938/1958, p. 135). Artaud attributes materiality to the affective world of the actor, and it is this materiality that he privileges over the seemingly psychological basis of words.

In his quest to access being or that which transcends the lack of being of the subject, the modality of performance is a means to invoke affect through the body and thereby access a certain truth beyond words. But what exactly is affect? I mentioned earlier that Damasio (1994) refers to Descartes' error as ignoring the role of feeling in rationality. Is feeling the same thing as affect? Not exactly, though Damasio does not clearly distinguish them in this text. I find that affect is very difficult to define satisfactorily, in terms of distinguishing emotion, feeling, and bodily sensation, and in many instances, they are generally grouped as affective responses. In *The Book of Love and Pain,* Juan David Nasio (2004) aligns pain with affect and argues that affect is a signifier, creating a very interesting link between feeling and the unconscious. Indeed, Soler (2016) points out the ambiguity of the word, as 'affect' relates to both the body and the subject, but its significance lies in the meaning of being affected by something. When we experience happiness, sadness, or anxiety, we are affected by it, and a valence is attached to the feeling or sensation. For Artaud, affect, as a feeling with a bodily component, or a sensation of the body that causes feeling, is also related to jouissance, a sense of a 'too muchness' in the body. What is this experience of excessive enjoyment if not, at some level, affect? Not all affect is jouissance but surely jouissance has to be affective. Indeed, John Dall'Aglio (2024) aligns jouissance with affective consciousness as a surplus of prediction error, where affect indicates something that needs to be addressed at the level of the drives. As Mark Solms puts it, affect tells us how we are doing in life—it is a benchmark of whether things are going well or badly (2021, p. 1069). Although the Lacanian view is that affects lie, I do not think this means we relegate them to a mystical ontological plane. Affects may displace and refer to a polyvalence of meaning rather than a singular truth but they may still be signifying and important. We are certainly affected by jouissance, which can be both within and outside of signification—for example, there is the jouissance of sense and the Other jouissance or so-called feminine jouissance, which is outside of the symbolic. To put it simply, I argue that, for Artaud, pain was a form of suffering but also a jouissance, a means of marking a limit in the body, a limit he wished to transgress and also to bring to bear through extremes of pleasure and pain. Attributing a limit to the body can ground the subject in a sense of being. A question may arise as to whether the pain I am speaking of is physical or mental, and in Artaud's case, it is both. We just need to take his opium addiction as an example, with the withdrawal symptoms that would have been felt at the level of the organic body as well as the mind, in terms of craving and the psychological ramifications of being addicted to a substance.

In an analysis of Artaud's later work, Chiesa (2006) argues that Artaud attempts to mediate the split of mind (as thought) and body (as materiality) through pain. I would add that at this point in Artaud's work, being becomes identified with suffering, and pain is the *affectual* mediator of the lack in being which has been "stolen by God" (2006, p. 348). But why is pain affect? We have already seen that for Freud, pain is a signal of the body's interiority or surface (a feeling of damage/wounding) and can overwhelm the rational mind; it is, to a certain extent, outside language. Pain is a breach of the ego defences—it undermines narcissistic mastery. If we take a neuropsychoanalytic view, affect is already a prediction error at the level of consciousness and we could say pain is an excess of this error—we *feel* pain, we don't *think* we are in pain. Given that affect (and the intensity of sensation or emotion) has a physical component, such as crying, laughing, and so on, and physical sensation is often aligned with immediacy, affect could be conceived as a vehicle to bridge the gap between thought and a more primal bodily form of experience. In other words, affect, deemed to be a sign of authenticity or truth, could be perceived as closer to being than thought.

In effect, for Artaud, then, pain (as bodily affect[3]) is potentially the mediator for arriving at some original point of 'satisfaction' (if being is aligned with suffering), where loss is transmuted into a libidinal presence of pain (as jouissance). As Chiesa notes:

> In 1946, shortly after his release, Artaud affirms: "I am there [*là*], / there means pain… I am there where I suffer. Being is suffering: in order to be, one has "to suffer being, all of being." Suffering, the immediacy of pain, which leaves the false dichotomy between the corporeal and the mental aside, becomes the sole and most immediate proof of my being real. It is in this sense that pain overlaps with the "purest reality", as Artaud had called it in *The Nerve Meter*: "This douleur driven into me like a wedge at the centre of my purest reality, at that region of sensibility where the two worlds of body and mind come together."
>
> (2006, p. 348)

If Artaud perceives that an authentic douleur has been stolen by God, this implies that he thought it possible to replace it, rather than remain lost as a structural metaphysical cause of existence. However, if, according to Lacan, affect cannot be being "in its immediacy nor is it the subject in a raw form either" (Lacan, 1962–1963/2014, p. 3), and we accept that pain is affect, then accessing being through pain is impossible. That affect is not the subject in a "raw form" indicates that affect may not be a superior form of 'knowing' concerning the subject and the body. In other words, a source of originality (as true meaning) may not be found in affect if indeed there is any origin concerning the subject. As Colette Soler (2016) argues, affect is not necessarily synonymous with truth, nor can it be separated from language:

> Whether experienced as a disruption of bodily homeostasis or experienced subjectively as a feeling that is more or less painful, affects are always so convincing to us that we are sorely tempted to mistake them for truth.
>
> (2016, p. 2)

As Artaud attempts to move away from the less 'authentic' expression of words and cognitive psychological understanding, he demonstrates a concern with the avoidance of repetition and the transcendent endeavour of achieving self-presence, as an essential originality. Interestingly, despite Artaud's insistence on originality, Bersani identifies a contradiction in Artaud's resistance to repetition, stating that Artaud "continuously repeats the project of abolishing repetitions" (2004, p. 98). Ironically then, the aspiration for originality is overshadowed by repeating the attempt to become original.

Artaud's project of transcending the psychologising/rational domain of the mind through corporeal theatre has important implications for thinking about contemporary idealisations of the body, including those in the therapeutic realm. These idealisations involve viewing the body as a source of truth, a container of traumatic memories to be released, and, in spiritual practices like yoga, a means of achieving transcendence of dividedness. In his manifesto for a Theatre of Cruelty, Artaud imagines a theatre that could release the repression of the unconscious through a bombardment of affect and sensation, an intensity of experience that could paralyse the mind (and hence his emphasis on psychological interpretations).

> In the true theatre a play disturbs the senses' repose, frees the repressed unconscious, incites a kind of virtual revolt (which moreover can have its full effect only if it remains virtual), and imposes on the assembled collectivity an attitude that is both difficult and heroic.
>
> (1938/1958, p. 28)

While I agree that theatre has the potential to challenge normative and ideological crystallisations inherent to the spectator's identity, I would question whether it can offer transcendence and freedom from unconscious repression. Not least because psychoanalysis demonstrates that physical catharsis or jouissance (as Artaud might have imagined it in performance) is not privileged over language in the release or uncovering of repression. As Bruce Fink (2019) argued in reference to the process of "affect hunting" in contemporary psychotherapy: affect hunting being the inclination to root out an intensity of feeling as a sign of authenticity, "It is only when thought and affect are brought together that repression can be overcome." In other words, repression cannot be undone or worked through simply by promoting affect alone. From this perspective, Artaud's project of transcending language by privileging the body as the vehicle for other modes of signification pertaining to affective response in the spectator does not seem possible. Language is always implicated in affect; words and signifiers *affect* us, they are connected to thoughts that generate feelings, or are connected to feelings. Futhermore, although affect may incur a certain sensation of immediacy, does this imply an immanence of being or does it really bring us knowledge of the body?

Given the impact of the signifier on the body and its relation to affect, language and speech inject space and distance into our experience of subjectivity. As soon as we speak of the body or try to represent it to somebody else, it becomes a signifier in a temporal sequence, something that is never quite what we were feeling. Pain can be a means of reducing a sense of distance between being the body. In states of severe pain, illness, or mental distress, the boundaries of inside and outside the subject can collapse, and the world outside the body shrinks to the more localised affect of pain, often creating an intensity of self-presence. Yet we can also lose touch with our bodies in these states. Admittedly, this is an abstract idea but one I have noticed in my own life. One is not necessarily more 'in touch' with one's body, and therefore present because of pain and the pressing necessity of biological contingency when things go awry in the body. In other words, affect is not necessarily the route to the being of the body and, hence, to a greater sense of authenticity. However, it can seem as if pain is a path to experiencing liberation from the ego or to unravel the self, as it is a humbling experience due to what we might imagine, in Freudian terms, to be a weakening of ego cathexis as a consequence of the flooding of the psyche with overwhelming affect. Suffering in any form, in fact, can challenge the narcissistic fantasies of wholeness and immunity to injury. The state of physical intensity and the lack of conscious thought often associated with pain is possibly what drove Artaud to privilege pain and bodily sensation as a vehicle for experiencing originality, a way of 'feeling' oneself acutely. Indeed, as Lacan, in *Seminar IX, Identification*, explains, pain can become a fetish given its propensity for taking over the body as libidinal affect:

> The experience of one pain effaces that of another, I mean that in the present it is difficult to suffer two pains at the same time: one takes over, makes one forget the other as if the libidinal cathexis, even onto one's own body, showed itself in this case to be subject to the same law which I would call that of partiality which motivates the relation to the world of the objects of desire.
>
> (Lesson XI, 22 February 1961–1962, p. 104)

It is clear that the body was undoubtedly a source of pain and conflict for Artaud. He was born with spinal meningitis and developed other physical afflictions over his lifetime, including opium addiction and other somatic symptoms, possibly in part due to psychosis.[4] From his writings, his work is not simply art as a representation of the conflict inherent to his experience but also an attempt to solve this bodily and metaphysical alienation and the invasive jouissance engendered by language. There is an inherent ambivalence in his writings regarding language. On the one hand, he attempts to transcend linguistic representation with other modes of theatrical signification. On the other, he writes copiously as if writing could suture the hole in being he circumvents with art. Through the actuality of the body on stage, mimesis as the distance inscribed within representation could become immanence, an immediacy of being. The Artaudian spectacle, such as it is comprised of gesture, movement, vocal invocations, envisages a performative form of representation that challenges Aristotle's definition of mimesis as imitation (Lehmann, 2006). The Artaudian spectacle does not endeavour to copy or imitate something but rather to be that something as transcendent presence and to capture the 'the in-itself' of embodied experience.

In terms of mind–body narratives, Artaud's project of reinventing the body through a language of corporeal signs was, in part, an idealisation of the body as a source of the truth of being and, in a sense, impossible. By aligning pain, cruelty, affect, and jouissance, it is possible to understand both Artaud's aesthetic of performance and his attempt to address a discordance at the levels of the body and of thought, as both a means of healing a Cartesian split and, strangely, affirming it. In the next chapter, we will look more closely at why his project to liberate the spectator from the unconscious through a bodily encounter with performance is problematic through an analysis of his only full-length staged play, *The Cenci.*

## Notes

1 Throughout the course of his life, Artaud made attempts to detox from opium but never succeeded in really quitting this substance. Stephen Barber (2003) notes in his biography of Artaud that opium featured significantly in his life and Artaud was demanding it while incarcerated in a mental hospital toward the end of his life. It is thus worth considering how opium, with its particular mode of toxic administration, its particularities of bodily and psychic effects may have operated as a sedative for a jouissance or suffering that Artaud simply couldn't bear. Within the context of Artaud's psychotic episodes, opium may have had a more complex stabilising function, quietening down the invasive presence of the Other. Of course, the addiction then created its own suffering, its own pain, the pain of withdrawal and the inability to tolerate reality without the substance. Furthermore, if we are to think of Artaud as an addicted subject, we develop a greater understanding of his position vis-à-vis the symbolic order, the realm of language and the social bond. Addicts have an ambivalent relationship to the Other. As Rik Loose (2002) argues in *The Subject of Addiction*, the substance nullifies a need for the social bond, seemingly causing an independence of sorts, but also keeps the subject dependent on an object, usually with underlying issues of insecure attachment and trauma.

2 Artaud's position on the unconscious is ambiguous. According to Murray (2014, p. 4), "Artaud was not interested in the unconscious, but in conscious thought as it emerged from and was mediated through the body, and he had no time at all for Surrealist practices such as automatic writing." However, I think Artaud was interested in the unconscious as he references it on various occasions in ways that show an awareness and great insight into its existence. Even his remark in The Theatre of Cruelty First Manifesto that language should have the effect it has in dreams indicates Artaud's interest in the realm beyond the conscious mind. He may not have wanted to accept the division that the unconscious represents but that is not the same thing as not being interested.

3 In *The Book of Love and Pain* (2004), Nasio places pain in the realm of affect and situates it as a phenomenon that goes beyond the pleasure principle: "Pain is an affect that reflects the extreme variation of unconscious tension in consciousness, variations that evade the pleasure principle" (p. 16).

4 In *Mad Like Artaud* (2003/2015), Sylvère Lotringer recounts that in 1938, Jacques Lacan examined Artaud in the psychiatric institution of the Sainte-Anne hospital in Paris and pronounced that he was fixed in his delusion and "will never write again." Lacan was clearly wrong in this pronouncement about Artaud's future as a writer, as the "mad poet" went on to write texts that would fill 25 volumes of the complete works (p. 39).

## References

Aristotle. (c.335 BC, 1996). *The poetics.* (M. Heath, Transl.) London: Penguin Books. https://disabilityarts.online/magazine/opinion/disability-a-creative-advantage/.

Artaud, A. (1938/1958). *The theatre and its double* (M.C. Richards, Transl.). New York: Grove Press.

Artaud, A. (1976). *Selected writings* (Ed. by S. Sontag. Transl. by H. Weaver & D. E. Levine). Farrar, Straus and Giroux.

Barber, S. (2003). *Blows and bombs. Antonin Artaud: The biography.* Creation books

Bersani, L. (2004). Artaud, defecation and birth. In E. Scheer (Ed.), *Antonin Artaud: A critical reader* (pp. 96–115). Routledge.

Chiesa, L. (2006). *Lacan: The silent partners* edited by Zizek. London and New York: Verso Books.

Chiesa, L. (2007). *Subjectivity and otherness: A philosophical reading of Lacan.* MIT Press.

Dall'Aglio, J. (2024). *A Lacanian neuropsychoanalysis: Consciousness enjoying uncertainty.* Palgrave Macmillan.

Damasio, A. (1994). *Descartes' error: Emotion, reason and the human brain.* Avon Books.

Elam, K. (2005). *The semiotics of theatre and drama.* Routledge.

Fink, B. (2019, May). *What is Lacanian psychoanalysis?* Presentation Dublin: APPI Conference.

Lacan, J. (1961–1962). *The seminar of Jacques Lacan. Book IX: Identification.* Unpublished. Cormac Gallagher.

Leader, D. (2001). *Jouissance: Sexuality, suffering and satisfaction.* Polity.

Lehmann, H.-T. (2006). *Postdramatic theatre.* Oxon: Routledge.

Loose, R. (2002). *The subject of addiction: Psychoanalysis and the administration of enjoyment.* Karnac.

Lotringer, S. (2015) *Mad like Artaud.* Transl. by Joanna Spinks. Univocal Publishing.

Morfee, A. (2005). *Antonin Artaud's writing bodies.* Oxford: OUP.

Murray, R. (2014). *The scum of the soul.* Palgrave Macmillan.

Nasio, J.D. (2004). *The book of love and pain.* New York: SUNY.

Rogers, A. (2016). *Incandescent alphabets: Psychosis and the enigmas of language.* Karnac.

Soler, C. (2016). *Lacanian affects: The function of affect in Lacan's work.* Transl. by B. Fink. Routledge.

Solms, M. (2021). Revision of drive theory. *Journal of the American Psychoanalytic Association*, 69 (6), 1033–1091. doi:10.1177/00030651211057041.

Turri, M.G. (2015). Transference and katharsis, Freud to Aristotle. *International Journal of Psychoanalysis*, 96, 369–387.

Chapter 7

# Theatre of Excess

## Modes of Jouissance in Artaud's *The Cenci*

Artaud's vision of a Theatre of Cruelty was brought to life in only one fully staged example, *The Cenci*. While Artaud's theoretical work gives voice to the trauma of the body as the impetus to repair or suture the discordance between body and mind, and is manifest in the construct of an impossible project or impossible body, tracing this phenomenon on stage is more difficult. This is partly because there is a gap between Artaud's theory of the Theatre of Cruelty, what he wanted to achieve and the reality of its staging, but also because working with the concept of ontological trauma is, by its very nature, hard to capture. In that sense, it is not simply through tangible representation that we can approach the trauma of the body, as this is structurally impossible; rather, trauma and the experience of conflict as regards the body are a driving force in the construction of the play's structure, plot, and narrative. While trauma as a narrative features strongly within the play through the themes of incest, violence, murder, parricide, and torture, these are somewhat contingent traumas rather than ontological—that is, what is contingent is also related to the ontological. However, from the perspective of the Theatre of Cruelty, it is through the performative work of these devastations that Artaud attempts to reform the bodily component of being by shattering the defences of the audience and exposing them to the potential horrors of life.

*The Cenci* was staged in 1935 at the Theatre des Folies-Wagram in Paris. This was Artaud's last theatrical production, in which he also acted in the role of the main protagonist, Count Cenci. The play was a disappointment from both a critical and a commercial point of view (Vork, 2013), but, as Vork points out, this lack of popular enthusiasm might have indicated success given its thematic content. *The Cenci* was brought to a close after 17 performances due to a lack of interest. Apart from the reviews that criticise Artaud's acting and the general format of the play, it is possible that the lack of enthusiasm is partly due to the subject matter concerned, that of incest and parricide. Despite the mixed reviews of *The Cenci*, a member of the audience summed up its import and spirit of invention as: "One can either love or detest this unusual play, but one should not remain indifferent to the

DOI: 10.4324/9781003509622-10

courage and audacity of the effort. (Blin, 1972, p. 40). For Artaud's only main play to be staged in full, its content is shocking, provocative, and indeed cruel on many levels. Artaud's production is loosely based on the true story of the Cenci family in sixteenth-century Italy, which has attained legendary significance, and is adapted from Percy Bysshe Shelley's verse form of the tragedy *The Cenci* (although Artaud claimed that this was an original play). The dramatisation of the Cenci family's downfall is one of horror and tragedy, with echoes of the Oedipal myth concerning parricide and incest.

Count Cenci is the main protagonist of the narrative and is a villain par excellence. Married to Lucretia, he is a father to four sons and one daughter, Beatrice. His ultimate aim is to control and dominate his whole family, and from the beginning of the play, Cenci makes these omnipotent intentions clear. He desires to exercise a supreme will over his family by murdering two of his sons and raping his daughter. Cenci succeeds in executing these acts, and subsequently, his traumatised and devastated daughter Beatrice plots revenge upon him, with the help of her mother and brother, by organising his murder by two mute assassins. She is then found guilty of executing this crime and, on papal orders, is sentenced to death, all the while refusing to admit or repent for her act. In this act of non-compliance unto death, her fate resembles that of Antigone, daughter of Oedipus, whose refusal to relent on her position regarding her brother's burial causes her own demise at the hands of her uncle, King Creon. In Lacan's *Seminar VII, The Ethics of Psychoanalysis,* Antigone's act of refusal and her uncompromising desire to bury her brother signify an ideal image of desire as manifest in the beauty of her tragic image. In this seminar, Lacan argues that the only thing one is guilty of is giving ground relative to one's desire (1959–1960, p. 321). One interpretation of this statement is that the blind determination to *not* give up on one's desire is the ideal ethical act, in which case anything goes as long as it is what you desire. However, the caveat to this interpretation is that desire is not straightforwardly deciphered; what we desire is often the Other's desire, manifest as something we are either rebelling against or conforming to. In *The Cenci,* Beatrice's stance toward her own death is equally staunch and self-sacrificing, although admittedly, the preceding incestuous trauma can be viewed as more immediate, more panic-stricken than Antigone's symbolic refusal to adhere to the law. Beatrice will not give up on her desire to oppose her father, even after his death, by capitulating and succumbing to the Pope's request for repentance. In this sense, Beatrice's act of non-compliance can be viewed from multiple perspectives and raises the following questions: is her non-capitulation to the admission of parricide an act of heroic and moral courage in the face of the abuse and injustice she has suffered at the hands of her father? Or is it a compulsion to repeat a morbid jouissance leading to her own death, a sign of her identification with her father? As her last line of the play poignantly reads: "In the end, I fear it will teach me I am not unlike him after all" (Artaud, 1935, 4.3. p. 153).

The position of Beatrice as a tragic heroine who avenges the incest she suffered can be contrasted with that of Dinah in Marina Carr's *On Raftery's Hill* (2000), an intensely brilliant and profoundly disturbing play where the trauma of incest permeates several generations of the Raftery family. Dinah's response to the abuse inflicted on her by her father is in stark contrast to Beatrice's radical confrontation of her abuser. This contrasting positioning gives a comparative lens to highlight the subjective responses to trauma. The trauma of abuse and the internal trauma of the drive[1] are always singular in how they are experienced (in that people are impacted differently and make individual choices in the face of the drive) and incorporate an ethical position regarding desire.

As a play concerned with the themes of incest and parricide, *The Cenci* is situated within the lineage of the historical and theatrical echoes of the Oedipal myth, as staged in one of Western literature's most significant tragedies, *Oedipus Rex* by Sophocles. Freud's theory of the Oedipus complex is loosely based on this myth and on Sophocles' version of the play. Originally, Freud postulated that a child unconsciously desires the parent of the opposite sex and becomes rivalrous with the parent of the same gender as themselves. However, in light of a reading of the Sophoclean tragedy, it is curious that, as Lacan (1959–1960) points out, Oedipus himself does not suffer from the Oedipus complex, as he slept with his mother and killed his father without knowing it. Freud contended that the Oedipal myth has provoked such fascination across the centuries because of its universal structure of human subjectivity. In other words, its widespread appeal was a testament to the representation of a fundamental desire of the human psyche and the relationship of the individual to the incest taboo. While the story of Oedipus is more prominently concerned with the desire of the child regarding the law against incest, in contrast to the transgression of the Father in *The Cenci,* it cannot be forgotten that it was King Laius who abandoned his son and left him to die. Therefore, the first sin of the Oedipal myth is that of the father's abandonment.

In contrast to the transgression of the incest taboo by the offspring in *Oedipus Rex,* in *The Cenci,* the father desires to violate his daughter and surpass the limits imposed by the symbolic order against this act. Count Cenci is a father who has no desire to control his destructive, abusive urges and expresses no remorse for these acts; he acts knowingly, without the ignorance of Oedipus. In his megalomania and fantasies of omnipotence, Count Cenci is comparable to the tyrannical father of the mythical primal horde, who has access to the All of jouissance and seeks to surpass the castration imposed by the law (Dempsey, 2012, p. 885). The myth of the primal father describes an imaginary state of existence preceding the law, before any limits were set, and before prohibition had been inculcated as a regulatory force. In this myth, the sons murder the father, and thus, the structures of modern civilisation are set in motion; the bonds of society are founded upon an act of destruction. The murder of the father is the act that triggers guilt, repression, and prohibition. Similarly, in Sophocles' play, Oedipus' recognition that he has married his mother and killed his father proves catastrophic and leads to his tragic downfall.[2] The guilt is too much to bear for Oedipus as he blinds himself with his mother's brooch after she hangs herself in horror at the realisation of her act. Oedipus recoils at the Real of his own drive and his ignorance of fulfilling the prophecy he tried to avoid. In this sense, the confrontation with the consequences of his own sexual drive becomes traumatic *after* realising that Jocasta is his mother.

In *The Cenci,* there is no such ignorance at work in the count's depraved lust; the forces of repression and conscience do not appear to operate in his character. In contrast to Oedipus' more neurotic, guilt-laden position vis-à-vis his incestuous act, he feels no guilt for his depraved desire. He would rather explain the causes of his deeds through fate and avoid taking responsibility: "Before anyone condemns my crime, let them accuse fate. Are we free? Who can maintain we are free when the heavens are ready to fall on us?" (Artaud, 1935/1974, p. 144). I said earlier that it was significant that Artaud played the role of Count Cenci, as I think we can trace Artaud's desire to transgress the law of the symbolic through this figure of megalomaniacal perversion. Could we postulate an aspiration for the twisted freedom inherent in someone who feels no guilt for raping his daughter and murdering his sons? Is this another image of an ideal of not giving up on one's desire? Or is Artaud intent on destroying the sacred position of the family within the kinship structures of society? We must remember that Artaud wanted to provoke the audience with the brute facts of life, that the sky may fall on our heads and that we are not free in many ways from the arrows of contingent circumstance. These lines appear in *The Cenci* and *The Spurt of Blood* (1925). That circumstances can be cruel does not simply mean the sky falling on our heads through a natural disaster or contingent event; it is often the case that horror occurs in the most familiar and intimate of social scenarios, namely, the family system.

In *The Cenci*, Artaud foregrounds the family unit as the source of extreme ill and wrongdoing. As he said, he wanted to challenge the myths associated with the family, what he refers to as its social superstition:

> In this play, nothing is treated with respect. I want to make everyone understand that I attack the social superstition of the family without asking one take up arms against such and such an individual. The same for order, same for Justice.
>
> (Artaud, 1935/1972, p. 92)

In treating nothing with respect and depicting the collapse of a nuclear family, Artaud attacks the fundamental structures supporting society, particularly by demonstrating a transgression of the taboo of incest, the ultimate destroyer of kinship structure. *The Cenci* inculcates disorder on a grand scale, from the microstructure of the family to the broader political and social context of the Church and the law. Count Cenci refuses to recognise any authority, and, in a sense, Beatrice does too. Artaud argues that the play is not an incitement to absolute anarchy but instead challenges the concept of order itself. In a Catholic context, the ideal of the heterosexual family is the bedrock of societal order, and its privileged place is protected by the dictates of the Catholic Church, headed by the Pope as master of the patriarchy. The concept of the nuclear family is founded on an ideal, as evidenced by all the attempts to protect this social unit from influences that would disrupt its very basis, such as contraception, homosexuality, incest, and infidelity. From a psychoanalytic perspective, the family can be viewed as a nexus of relations founded upon the repression of the drive toward Oneness, a state of blissful undifferentiatedness encapsulated by the unity of the mother and child, which exists before the separating and alienating effects of language have taken place. From this perspective, we could say that Artaud's version of the play (as performed in the style of the Theatre of Cruelty) attempts to undo the forces of repression and to generate the jouissance of transgressing the law. We must also remember that the impulse to symptomatic jouissance is often a means of attempting to quell a more difficult primary form of jouissance, possibly in the form of bodily (somatic) suffering. In other words, jouissance, as that enjoyment of the body or pleasure in pain, exists on different levels. It is often both a release and a cause of suffering. In *The Cenci,* this quest for what Vork calls "annihilation" reaches its zenith with the actions of a villain whose mode of jouissance disobeys any form of societal or mythical loss.

In the figure of the Count, the play stages a terrifying confrontation with a form of enjoyment that exceeds the law and the symbolic order. Count Cenci's mode of jouissance is devouring and cannibalistic (characteristic of the oral drive) and features a will to incorporate into himself all that he has procreated, to leave no space from which his children can separate from him. Trauma is a systemic theme in this drama and can be approached both structurally and narratively as something performed through the interplay of presence and absence, language and the unspoken. It is something obviously embedded within the heinous acts, that is, within the horror that is provoked in the spectator, but it is also inferred through the pre-emptive nature of the rape and Beatrice's anxiety in advance. The anticipation of a horrific event is illustrated by Beatrice's knowledge that her father intends to rape her as he makes it clear to her that this is what he intends to do. The staging of the premeditated nature of Count Cenci's rape is particularly grotesque, even more so (if it is possible to say) than a seemingly impulsive act of sexual assault. From the perspective of the performance's particularities, and in keeping with Stendhal's style, Vork explains that these 'unspeakable acts' are never actually depicted in Artaud's production. Instead, they take place between the spaces in the acts and dialogue and are referred to as "acts" or "actions." (2013, p. 313). This technique contrasts with the violence portrayed in Carr's play, where at the end of the first act, the spectator is confronted with the horror of the incestuous act as the father rapes his youngest daughter, Sorel, on the kitchen table. The full brutal spectacle of this scene, which contrasts with that of *The Cenci* (as we don't actually see the rape of Beatrice), has the effect of incorporating the spectator's desire as a passive onlooker of this depravity. Sorel asks us for help, and we sit idly by. This provocation is evocative of the reality of the experience of abuse and incest sufferers, and the disbelief and disapproval they can encounter in those to whom they have confided their experience.

## Beyond the Law: Cenci and Beatrice

In *The Cenci,* destruction is at the apex of the acts committed. As Artaud states: "The father in *The Cenci* is a destroyer. And it is in such a way that this subject revives the Great Myth" (Blin, 1935/1972, p. 16). Although Artaud doesn't specify, the reference to the Great Myth here may be a reference to the father of the primal horde, or that of Oedipus Rex. In Act One, Scene 1, Count Cenci's destructive impulse is expressed in flagrantly candid terms:

> There is no life, no death, no God, no incest, no contrition, no crime in my existence. I obey my own law, of which I am my own master … My rule, my intent, is to seek out and to practice evil. I cannot resist the forces burning with violence inside me.
>
> (Artaud, 1935/1974, 1.1, p. 123)

Furthermore, he outlines the particularity of the pleasure associated with evil: "Evil, after all, is not without its pleasures. I shall torture the soul while enjoying the body." (Artaud, 1935/1974, 1.1, p. 124). Thus, Count Cenci gives voice to a state of division between body and soul concerning a certain enjoyment of the body, an excess of the flesh. Through the desire to dominate and subvert the law of the social order, the Count releases the aggressive, sadistic impulse of the drive.

The acts committed by Count Cenci exceed any rational argument; he makes no excuses for his pursuit of jouissance. In this context, his acts are in the Real; there is no accounting for them, and they go beyond the law of the social order, a law that prohibits incest. Cenci wants to embody his own law, a law that destroys as the ultimate power and that has no investment in the symbolic order.

CENCI: There can be no human relationships between those born only to replace their kin, between those thirsting to devour one another.

LUCRETIA: But there would be no society if such ideas were true.
CENCI: The family I command and that I have created is the only society I recognise.
LUCRETIA: That is tyranny.
CENCI: Tyranny is my last remaining weapon to fight your war against me.
(Artaud, 1935/1974, p. 134)

Thus, tyrannical and despotic, Cenci defies any obstacle to his satisfaction and is a horrifying portrait of the desire to become One (like the primal father, omitting all lack) in relation to an enjoyment of the flesh. While the central figure of depravity, the modalities of jouissance in the play go beyond those illustrated by the deranged father. The position of Beatrice's desire toward the murder of her father and her own impending death is also crucial in this analysis.

Although Beatrice's story and fate are inherently tragic, in technical terms, she may not qualify as a tragic heroine, given that she does not reach a point of anagnorisis in the play (Dempsey, 2012, p. 880). She does not admit the truth of her action and refuses to accept responsibility, continually stating her innocence up to the end, despite her torture in prison. However, in another light, this recalcitrance regarding her crime can also be understood as a stubborn refusal to capitulate to her father even after he has died. A confession would admit defeat, but her battle cry is motivated by a plea for just revenge: how can there be murder when her father has committed such a heinous violation? Beatrice, like Antigone, does not refuse to cede to her desire; she holds steadfast despite knowing she will die. Although she may not be a tragic heroine, her character has an ethical dimension, and her choices determine her fate. Despite her protests of innocence, Beatrice is not without feelings of ambivalence towards her abuser: "I ought to hate him, yet I cannot. His living form is inside me like the guilt of a crime" (Artaud, 1935/1974, p. 132). Again, like Antigone, who awaits her own death in the cave, lamenting the life not led and grieving her demise, Beatrice also regrets the losses incurred in her untimely exit. As she laments:

> I am to die, yet I have not chosen to do so […] to die so young. To be swallowed by the mournful earth, endlessly cursing oneself. The world I leave behind will not survive me […] My heart was never happy, yet it will stop beating before it has ever been stirred.
>
> (Artaud, 1935/1974, p. 153)

Artaud's portrayal of Beatrice as the recalcitrant heroine would seem to have echoes with that of the fate of Antigone. Indeed, Antigone's staunch position clearly resonated with Artaud and in a text entitled *Antigone chez les Francais* (1977), written while interred in Rodez, Artaud recounts the power of Antigone's name as a legacy and inspirational force in the battle of the self against the forces of being: "Antigone est le nom de cette victoire terrible..." (p. 154). For Lacan also, Antigone signified an image of tremendous resistance in the face of the desire of the Other, and her intransigent position toward her uncle, Creon, made her a heroine or an exemplar of sorts for the process of psychoanalysis. Lacan's argument in *Seminar VII* on the image of Antigone and how something of the tragic dimension of desire is transmitted to the spectator is fascinating from the perspective of the dialectic between psychoanalysis and artworks.[3] We will return to the function of the image within the structure of the drama shortly, when considering how Artaud attempts to jolt the spectator out of complacency or to move their perception beyond the realm of the imaginary. One way of doing this was, as he said in the *Theatre and Its Double*, to have language have the effect of a dream, to provoke the unconscious of the spectator. In *The Cenci*, dreaming forms part of the narrative structure and serves not only to provoke the spectator's unconscious but also to provide an entry into the complexities of Beatrice's trauma.

## Marking the Unspeakable: Beatrice's Dream

Artaud said that the characters in *The Cenci* say most of what they are thinking and also what they cannot say. As a signifier of the unconscious and of what cannot be spoken without censorship, dreams play an important role in the play's spoken and unspoken dialogue and dramatic architecture. Through an account of Beatrice's dream, we gain insight into her relationship to the traumatic 'knowledge' of her sexuality and her father's previous pursuit of her:

> When I was little, I had the same dream every night. I was naked, alone in a vast bedroom with a wild animal such as only exists in dreams. I could hear it breathing. I could escape, but I had to hide my glaring nudity.
>
> (Artaud, 1935/1974, p. 140)

Beatrice's dream, or rather, this nightmare, indicates her awareness regarding the danger surrounding her sexuality and the presence of a menacing force that pursues her. The fact that she dreamed this sequence of images "every night", or in other words, repeatedly, emphasises its traumatic dimension, displaying the repetition-compulsion inherent to its continuous manifestation. In the dream, Beatrice is aware that she can escape the danger by covering her body and nudity; her desire or wish to escape the wild animal resonates with her position in the play regarding her father's advances. Therefore, we get the impression that she has been sensing these wild animalistic forces (embodied by her father) pursuing her all her life, and consequently, her trauma extends far beyond the present circumstance. Freud said that dreams operated in the psyche as "the royal road to the unconscious", and in the case of traumatic neuroses, they served to enact, within the dream, the compulsion to repeat the painful, traumatic experience. In *The Interpretation of Dreams* (1900), Freud discussed the symbolism of wild beasts for the dreamer:

> The dream-work usually symbolises passionate impulses; those of the dreamer, and also those of other persons of whom the dreamer is afraid; or thus, by means of a very slight displacement, the persons who experience these passions. From this, it is not very far to the totemistic representation of the dreaded father by means of vicious animals, dogs, wild horses, etc. One might say that wild beasts serve to represent the *libido,* feared by the ego, and combated by repression.
>
> (Freud, 1900, p. 197)

In *Beyond the Pleasure Principle* (1920), Freud places the dreams of injured soldiers who relive the painful experiences as an example of that which exceeds the pleasure principle. In Beatrice's dream, the wild beast may be a symbolic representation of her father, but another facet to consider is that it is also a metaphor for her sexuality—that unruly, wild animal from which she attempts to escape. In this context, therefore, an image of a wild beast may represent an internal instinct, something that is innate to her yet pertains to the primitive realm, a metaphor for the sexual drives that threaten the ego with fragmentation and danger. It is also significant that the wild beasts are described in the plural: "there is not one beast, but many of them swarming at her feet" (Artaud, 1935/1974, p. 140).

That the forces pursuing Beatrice are also her own inner compulsions is illustrated through the implication of her singular subjective position in the language of the dream. In describing the thirst of the wild beasts, there is a slippage in Beatrice's reference to her thirst: "And this horde was also thirsty… I realised my thirst was not only stubbornness." (1935/1974, p. 140). This verbal slippage indicates that Beatrice is both separate from and included in the wild horde. Furthermore, the moment Beatrice wakes from this dream is of great significance and indicates the missed encounter with trauma as the Real that cannot be encountered. As she recounts: "Each time I felt my strength was about to fail, I immediately awoke" (1935/1974, p. 140). Instead of experiencing that horrifying moment where the beasts catch up with her, and she confronts 'the thing', Beatrice wakes up to (as the events in this play show), a reality more terrifying than that which the dream can signify.[4] It is at the very point of a trauma (the 'missed encounter') that cannot be represented in images or words that Beatrice wakes up, and her becoming conscious at this point serves as a cut that marks a rupture in the events. Her waking up at this moment of terror prevents an encounter with the void (Real) that would render her absent as a subject. In the waking moments of the play, with the advances of her father startlingly close, Beatrice recognises that life is a dream (or nightmare) from which there is no waking up, apart from through death. Vork accurately contends that just as the heinous acts committed are not depicted in actuality, the dream sequence in *The Cenci* functions to mark what cannot be presented, or represented concerning subjectivity within the performance structure of the play (2013, p. 318).

Interestingly, the feature of the dream is a detail introduced by Artaud into the plot structure, an addition to Shelley's rendition and demonstrates Artaud's affiliation with the surrealists and his interest in the unconscious. The inscriptions of the dream index a metaphysical space (the unconscious) where representation fails within the performance as staged space and is an appropriation of the 'unsayable', where an event or feeling cannot be directly depicted. As we know from psychoanalysis, that which is repressed returns in dreams, in disguised form, serving partly to release the tension of the veiled wish or desire.

In the torture scene at the end of the play, Beatrice expresses the ambivalence she feels regarding her father and her fear of becoming just like him. This is the real tragedy of her act of parricide; her revenge has caused her to act brutally and to die with blood on her hands, resembling somewhat the crimes of her father. The tragic figure of Beatrice, like Antigone, may well have been an icon of heroism for Artaud. In *The Theatre and Its Double,* Artaud expresses a fascination with the character Annabella in *'Tis Pity She's a Whore* (*c.*1633) by John Ford, a character who bears a strong resemblance to Beatrice. Artaud writes:

> Annabella is captured, convicted of adultery and incest, trampled upon, insulted, dragged by the hair, and we are astonished to discover that far from seeking a means of escape, she provokes her executioner still further and sings out in a kind of obstinate heroism. It is the absolute condition of revolt; it is an exemplary case of love without respite which makes us, the spectators, gasp with anguish at the idea that nothing will ever be able to stop it.
>
> (Artaud, 1938/1958, p. 29)

Artaud wanted the spectator to truly feel, on a sensory level, the powerlessness of witnessing such a tragic fate. His emphasis on anguish as the affectual response he wanted the spectacle to generate is significant, as within Lacan's terminology, it is the one affect that doesn't lie (Soler, 2016), meaning that anguish leads us to a confrontation with the Real—it is a signal of traumatic enjoyment—where our subjectivity is most at stake.

## Performing Destruction: Beyond the Imaginary?

In directing the play, Artaud was categorical that the performance would incorporate his vision of a Theatre of Cruelty, namely that it would penetrate the nerves of the spectator and engage the senses. He writes:

> I want the theatrical representation to have the aspect of a devouring focus where action, situation, characters and images are brought to a degree of implacable incandescence: Through my play I also want the public to be plunged into a bath of fire... What happiness for me if I can make the spectator participate with his soul and his nerves in the tragedy of *The Cenci!*
>
> (Artaud quoted in Blin, 1972, p. 14)

The phrase 'devouring focus' is apt when considering the cannibalistic and devouring passion exhibited by Count Cenci, thereby revealing that the form and architecture of the performance reflect the narrative content. Artaud's vision of the spectacle would engulf the spectator in the form of an incandescent experience. He aligns theatrical representation with the cannibalistic quality of the oral drive, in which the elements of theatrical performance devour the participating audience members. The Theatre of Cruelty was designed to move from the static enactment of staging verisimilitude as a reflection of life toward a dynamic dialectic between actor and spectator. In speaking of the dynamics of character in *The Cenci,* Artaud writes: "This character who says what he thinks represents at the same time my own thought but represents it dramatically, that is to say dynamically, that is to say dialectically" (Artaud quoted in Blin, 1972, p. 92).

The dialectic that Artaud speaks of here is the extension of his own being through the dramatisation enacted by the characters, and in this particular case, we might imagine that Count Cenci activates at least some of his inner thoughts. Artaud's stress on the emphasis of tone and volume of sound and intensity of lighting in a theatrical production was an attempt to bypass (as sensory experience) what he felt to be the rationality of language and dialogue in Occidental theatre. In Artaud's words:

> Text, gesture, sound, lighting-each is equally important to me. The play lives off this whole, and whoever neglects one of these elements is depriving this body of an essential organ ... There is no true language in the theatre except action. It alone counts.
>
> (Artaud quoted in Blin, 1935/1972, p. 97)

In this passage, Artaud aligns the elements of the theatrical production with the organs of the body, or the play itself as being a body, an interesting precursor to his concept of the body without organs. The spectator in the Theatre of Cruelty should be set adrift from the everyday coordinates of social reality and its habitual moderations and cast into the flames that burn the body from within. In his artistic development, theory and ideas, Artaud was certainly visionary and inspiring; yet, as Jannarone (2010) argues, there was another side to this productive insistence that was nihilistic and tyrannical. It is certainly worth considering the motivation or the potentially narcissistic desire to bring the spectator to submission, as he puts it. Why is this so important for Artaud?

Jannarone is critical of Artaud's drive for complete control of the production, as his directing of the play displayed omnipotent didacticism and obsessive instructions. She says that, for all of Artaud's proclamations of anarchy, the staged directions are, ironically, more imbued with a genre of order, what she calls "organised anarchy" (p. 171). In this context of organisation, it is highly significant that Artaud chose to play the role of Count Cenci, the tyrannical, despotic Lord, which by certain accounts was viewed as an inappropriate casting. If we view it from Jannarone's perspective, Artaud's desire to control and dominate the spectator through the forces of the spectacle becomes realised in his embodiment of the despotic Cenci. Therefore, I would argue that, through the medium of theatre, Artaud transforms delusion into fantasy by taking something that exists for him at the level of the Real (non-meaning), such as the sexual non-rapport, and transmuting it onto the stage of illusion, thereby transforming the Real into fiction. Why indeed is this a fantasy? It would seem that the preoccupation with the spectator and generating affect is a means of making the Other exist in some way. Indeed, this Other is not lacking in the sense that Artaud intended for them to experience anguish and powerlessness, a sense of being at the mercy of fate. Although Artaud wanted to affect the Real in the spectator, enacting something within the theatre space also brings something unsaid or unsignified into the symbolic and the imaginary. It's as if he wanted to induce lack in the spectator, perhaps curtailing the invasive jouissance of an Other without limits.

The use of intense sound and lighting to evoke a visceral response in the audience is a technique that aims to break down the distance between the stage and the audience, acting on the nerves and body of the spectator. Thus, an Artaudian catharsis, as Laurens de Vos (2011) calls it, is one of a "too much" of the spectacle, and a surpassing of what may be tolerated comfortably, a theatrical enactment of a beyond of the pleasure principle, a jouissance of the senses. Or in Artaud's words, "Cruelty also acts against the spectator, and it must not permit him to leave the theatre intact, but he also must be exhausted, involved, transformed, perhaps!" (Artaud quoted in Blin, 1935/1972, p. 107)

The use of sound, in particular, in *The Cenci* is worth pausing to consider its role in Artaud's strategy of evoking the sensations of the body through bodily-related performance stimuli. The voice and its correlative sound are among the most enigmatic concepts in psychoanalysis, yet they allow us to consider how the body can extend itself beyond its physical frame. The body, in effect, is captured by the voice and sound can have a profound impact on the body. We can even think of the body as being composed of vibrational energetic pathways to which certain sounds respond. Artaud devised an intricate soundscape for *The Cenci*, which, Curtin argues (2010), was part of the means of activating the spectator's subconscious to purge repressed desires and ultimately render the person less likely to commit such acts in reality. The effect of sound was to operate on the audience as a means of unifying them and as the receptor of a hieroglyphic meaning, albeit communicated through a non-visual or linguistic medium. Curtin argues why this method may not have been effective in Artaud's intention and I think it speaks to a wider point about Artaud's invention of hieroglyphic communication, per se:

> Consequently, the sound design for Les Cenci could not elicit the hieroglyphic clarity, the 'direct seizure of transcendental knowledge', to which Artaud aimed, because the sounds it deployed probably multiplied or confounded meaning rather than 'spiritually' concentrating it.
>
> (2010, p. 256)

While believing somewhat in unconscious forces, indeed, Artaud's logic has been compared to an inversion of Lacan's famous adage that the unconscious is structured like a language, with his viewpoint being more "language is structured by the unconscious" (David Cooper quoted in Jay Murphy 2016), Artaud seems to take a somewhat universalising approach to the potential impact of theatre on the spectator. Whether this sensory provocation really has a transformative effect on the spectator is very debatable, as is what being transformed would look like. Can art or drama really change us? And what would this change signify? Is it a moment of realisation of our dividedness, a glimpse of the unconscious, that space of knowing of which we do not want to know? These are huge questions, and, in essence, in part, what I am trying to answer with this book, while hoping not to fall into an Artaudian impasse—that is, by trying to make the Real visible or symbolisable. There is something of the ontology of the body of which we are not conscious, but that can be provoked through art, psychoanalysis and theatre, even through the very failure to represent this traumatic corporeal ontology. Can theatre 'deform' the imaginary? — a question partly built on Chiesa's point that the ego-ideal can have a deformative effect on identification. Furthermore, only certain ego-ideal formations have the power to deform the ideal ego (2007, p. 39). That is to say, the primary narcissistic image that we have of ourselves is not that easily altered or transformed and may only become modified through primary and significant attachment objects. Nonetheless, works of art, novels, films, and dramatic performances (as part of the symbolic order) have the potential to influence the normative and preconceived conceptions of ourselves, even for a moment. Putting it differently, what we see can reorientate us to how we see ourselves, either in the form of an alienating rupture, what Olga Cox Cameron (2018) refers to as the knocking out of the imaginary through the spectacle of tragedy or by providing succour for our fantasies of fulfilment.

Similarly, Todd McGowan (2007) refers to the potential of a film to disrupt our ideological position regarding enjoyment, "in the trauma of the gaze lies the freedom of the subject" (p. 210). Another way of viewing this is that certain performances (or works of art) disrupt our habitual relationship to everyday objects of knowledge (including what we perceive as our own bodies) and provide possibilities for the dismantling of signifiers and signifieds.

So why is Artaud considered somewhat of a failed practitioner? I would say it is because there was a strong element of the impossible in what he was trying to do, and even if he succeeded in conveying this impact in words, it would, according to his logic, not be an adequate means of representation. We need to remember that part of what constitutes the body is its construction through language and the imaginary dimensions of images and identifications. It is not simply a physical substance that can be modified through sensory experiences.

From a more simplistic perspective, Artaud's theatre was designed to provoke the spectator into a more alive state than the numbing effect of simply engagement with a source of entertainment, an escape from the worries of the world, and in this sense his use of the great myths and the shocking themes of rape and incest are tapping into the primal horrors and seductions that exist for all of us and that threaten the cohesion of subjectivity and the social order. From the reviews of *The Cenci* after its staging in Paris, it is clear that people were certainly not indifferent; perhaps even negative reviews are signs that Artaud achieved, at least in part, his purpose.

Artaud's transcendental project cuts to the core of one of the questions I have about the possibility of theatre impacting us in such a way that the imaginary identifications that shield us from the reality of our incoherent selves are deformed, engendering a confrontation with the Real of experience. Or, in other words, can theatre, depending on the modality of performance, provide us with a glimpse of our fantasy structures that support the miscognitions of the body-mind identifications and the insistence on ableism as the only way of being in the modern world?

In seeking a theatrical performance that acts directly on the body, Artaud aims to disorient the spectator, to dislodge them from the presumptions and logic of the conventional symbolic order, and to create new forms of being through the language of gesture and the elements of mise-en-scène. This was why theatre was not a form of mimesis but a fully alive force that cultivates an awakened spectator who participates in the dramatic action with their very being. For the route to being for Artaud, as I have argued in the previous chapter, was that of the body. Being is opposed to thinking, or at least Artaud attempts to embody thought, bringing cognition to the level of the sensory. The question is whether a play like *The Cenci*, in its staged Theatre of Cruelty modalities, achieves this aim. Can impacting the body of the spectator through an affectual resonance of performance cause transformation, a breakdown in identifications that shield us from the Real of being and provoke insight into repression? In other words, can it break through the imaginary as the realm of misrecognition, ego-oriented knowledge, to nominate something in the Real? Is there such a thing as any linguistically unmediated impact on the body through the reception of stimuli through the senses? Can it in fact release repression and cause a liberation of tension? We need to remember that even when we are dealing with the sensory body, the imaginary comes into play in how senses are interpreted and managed by the psychic apparatus. In Artaud's logic, there appears to be a privileging of sensation and affect as if this could somehow be a purer experience, a route to unconscious knowledge. Even if this can be triggered in the spectator, what then occurs for a person after an experience of anguish may not be transformative in the way Artaud envisaged. For example, it could lead to shutting down or denial in a defensive reaction to the disturbance of anxiety. Artaud was against the psychologisation of events, or what we could call an interpretive account of affect, a moral distribution of cause and effect in action, a way of containing intense feeling through cognitive appraisal of relevant elements. In a way, Artaud's resistance to psychologisation is akin to exposing the imaginary dimension of subjectivity, that realm of seemingly rational yet internally awry perspectives that provide explanations while still remaining at the level of the ego or generalisations. There is quite a presumption on his part that, to put it very simply, he knows what is best for the spectator. For Artaud, the aim of theatre was not about simply staging make-believe but rather it endeavoured to make present what was already pertinent to the spectator's inner life, the drives of which the spectator may not be conscious. As he says:

> The spectator with the truthful precipitates of dreams, in which his taste for crime, his erotic obsessions, his savagery, his chimeras, his utopian sense of life and matter, even his cannibalism, pour out, on a level not counterfeit and illusory, but interior.
>
> (Artaud, 1938/1958, p. 92)

In writing about the spectators' predilections for horrific crimes and fantasies of destruction, Artaud was also writing about himself. This destruction is in part typified by the theme of incest as the ultimate perversion of the symbolic order and is found also in *The Spurt of Blood*. What was it about incest that so fascinated him?

## Incest as a Subversion of Sexuality

With the production of *The Cenci,* Artaud attacked and challenged the ideal of the heterosexual nuclear family, or as he referred to it, the "social superstition" of the family. In attacking the ideology of the family, Artaud could subvert the basis of order itself and formulate his own founding myth; he will eventually say that he is his own father and mother. According to various critical perspectives, Artaud was attempting to recreate a form of unity, a merging with the Real before division and the trauma of language cultivates us as speaking subjects. This is perhaps why he chooses one of the most pertinent subjects for tragedy historically, that of incest and parricide. In this subversion of order, the fundamental prerequisites for existing as a subject also come under attack, including sexuality and procreation. It was known amongst his friends and associates that Artaud found the idea of sex and procreation unpalatable. As Jannarone states, his theatre did not celebrate naked bodies but rather expressed "a loathing of the body and of sex" (2010, p. 15).

This loathing of the body and of sex indicates a profound anxiety in relation to sexuality. As Lotringer (2015) recounts in *Mad Like Artaud,* Artaud was terrified of women and particularly of pregnant women, spitting as he went past his psychiatrist's pregnant wife to avoid contact with demons. Although Artaud's position regarding his fear of women might have implied homosexuality, it is more likely that his horror of sexuality was a consequence of his relationship to meaning and the trauma of the desire of the Other. According to Lotringer, Artaud was almost certainly incapable of having sex. His drawings throughout his stay in the sanatorium of Rodez depict scenes of great fragmentation and death and images of copulation, suffering bodies and disembodied vaginas. Furthermore, Martin Esslin underlines a contradiction inherent to Artaud's relationship to sexuality. As he says, although Artaud "saw salvation in sexual excess and the wildest indulgence of the senses", he also saw sexuality as "the ultimate source of all the ills that beset mankind" (1976, p. 7).

In chapter 3, we saw that sexuality, per se, is traumatic for all human beings. The internal drives are hard to manage and leave us at the Other's mercy in satisfying our desires. There is no ultimate rapport between the sexes or for those of the same sex, so a gap always remains in how we are responded to. However, fantasy can provide a shield for the trauma of the Other's lack and love, as Lacan says, is what makes up for the lack in the sexual relation. For Artaud, fantasy does not seem to cover the hole in the Real and the relation to the object a was one of excess rather than absence—something to be enjoyed rather than desired, and the vicissitudes of sex and the mystery of procreation (symbolised by pregnant females, for example) constituted a trauma, a hole in his subjectivity. In this sense, sexuality may have been experienced as an acute manifestation of the death drive, a phenomenon that threatened to engulf his body through a jouissance that lacked the limits of the pleasure principle. He was driven to represent sexuality through fantasy and fiction as the real encounter, staged through the body of another person, was too traumatic. Language could not contain this oppressive force of the drive and the Theatre of Cruelty, designed to surpass language, was a necessary failure on the path to exceeding the limits of normative representation. While his corporeal theatre still retained some traces of the parameters of an earthly body, Artaud needed to invent another way of dealing with the trauma of the body and to reimagine its structure within the concept of an impossible entity: a body without organs. With this, he could redefine the parameters of being.

## Notes

1 I would qualify this by adding that the drive can be experienced as more disturbing because of trauma and the tearing of a hole in the ego's defensive or excitation managing qualities.
2 As Freud says, "His fate (Oedipus) moves us only because it might have been our own, because the oracle laid upon us before our birth the very curse which rested upon him. It may be that we were all destined to direct our first sexual impulses toward our mothers, and our first impulses of hatred and violence toward our fathers; our dreams convince us that we were. King Oedipus, who slew his father Laius and wedded his mother Jocasta, is nothing more or less than a wish-fulfilment—the fulfilment of the wish of our childhood." (Freud, 1900, p.110)
3 See Meehan O'Callaghan (2024), *Lacunae*, for a full discussion of this.
4 An example of trauma as an encounter with the Real in a dream is elaborated by Lacan through 'the dream of the burning child' in *The Four Fundamental Concepts of Psychoanalysis* (1964). In the father's dream, the child's reproach, "Father, can't you see I'm burning?" (p. 34), poses a question about the nature of what is being experienced as the Real.

## References

Artaud, A. (1974/1935). The Cenci (V. Corti, Transl.). In *Collected works* (Vol. 4). London: John Calder.

Artaud, A. (1938/1958). *The theatre and its double* (M.C. Richards, Transl.). New York: Grove Press.

Artaud, A. (1977). Antigone chez les français. In *Nouveaux ecrits de Rodez*. Gallimard.

Blin, R. A. (1972). Antonin Artaud in *Les Cenci. Drama Review*, 16 (2), June, 90–145.

Carr, M. (2018). *On Raftery's hill*. Staged at the Abbey Theatre, Dublin.

Cox Cameron, O. (2018). The worst is not while we can say: This is the worst. *Lacunae* (17), 50–74.

Curtin, A. (2010). Cruel vibrations: Sounding out Antonin Artaud's production of *Les Cenci. Theatre Research International*, 35, 250–262.

De Vos, L. (2011). *Cruelty and desire in the modern theatre: Antonin Artaud, Sarah Kane, and Samuel Beckett*. Kindle edition.

Dempsey, S. (2012). The Cenci: Tragedy in a secular age. *ELH*, 79 (4), 879–903.

Esslin, M. (1976). *Antonin Artaud: The man and his work*. Calder Publications.

Freud, S. (1900). *The interpretation of dreams*. Retrieved from www.abika.com.

Freud, S. (1920). *Beyond the pleasure principle*. (Authorised Translation from the 2nd German edition by C.J.M. Hubback). (E. Jones, Ed.) Rosings Digital Publications. Retrieved 25 August 2018.

Jannarone, K. (2010). *Artaud and his doubles.* University of Michigan Press.
Lacan, J. (1959–1960/1997). *Seminar VII. The ethics of psychoanalysis.* (J.-A. Miller, Ed., & D. Porter, Transl.) London: Norton & Company.
Lacan, J. (1964/1978). *The seminar of Jacques Lacan. The four fundamental concepts of psychoanalysis.* (J.-A. Miller, Ed., & A. Sheridan, Transl.) New York: Norton.
Lotringer, S. (2015) *Mad like Artaud.* Transl. by Joanna Spinks. Univocal Publishing.
Vork, R. (2013). Things that no one can say: The unspeakable act in Artaud's *Les Cenci. Modern Drama*, 56 (3), 306–326.

# Part III

# The Body Between Being and Non-Being

Part III of this book turns to a more detailed consideration of how the trauma of the body in Beckett and Artaud frames a question concerning being. For both authors, the body is not a stable entity but rather a question, something to be interrogated; or, to put it differently, the body is a route to pursuing a question of being, that which is most essential, most primordial about the existence of the human being.

This chapter and the next will elaborate on how both Beckett and Artaud, in different ways, engage with the phenomenon of being through the performative manipulation of the physical body and through the relationship to language inherent to their work. In Beckett's case, this discussion will focus on an actual performance, that of *Not I*; in Artaud's, in part, due to a dearth of staged theatrical performances but also the performativity of his later work in art, radio and writing, it will be more theoretically eclectic, drawing on his desire to invent a new body through the concept of the body without organs and offering an overview of the body's relation to being in contemporary contexts.

DOI: 10.4324/9781003509622-11

Chapter 8

# *Not I*: Delimiting the Void of Being

A mouth suspended in the dark, a voice unmoored from any body, *Not I* takes the spectator to the edge of an abyss, an abyss delimited by a human orifice suspended in space and shrouded by darkness. While *Endgame* (1958) revealed Beckett's aesthetic of debility through the incapacities of bodies within a moribund world, in *Not I* (1972), one of Beckett's later plays, the body comes under increasing erasure as a source of any stability of being. In this ultimate performance of Beckettian phenomenal subtraction, the motif of the absent body culminates in a form at once strange and too familiar. Through Mouth's uncanny form—an organ without a body—we enter a zone of aesthetic deformations where the reassuring landmarks of quotidian corporeal forms are absent. Instead, we are shrouded in the dark, at the mercy of a frantic voice and a mouth that symbolises the not whole body. In this stark rendition of a raving mind, a gaping mouth, only the lips and teeth visible, speaks at tremendous speed while a hooded auditor of "sex undeterminable" stands downstage raising arms occasionally "in a gesture of helpless compassion" (Beckett, 1972/2006, p. 375). There is no physical body attached to the mouth that we can see; it has been covered to magnify the presence of the deranged orifice that speaks as if from nowhere and to no one in particular. Actresses who have performed the part of Mouth, such as Billie Whitelaw and Lisa Dwan, were required to place their bodies in a restrictive posture on stage. The body was effectively tied in place so that the head and mouth would remain as still as possible, amplifying the oral orifice as a singular and autonomous body part. Lisa Dwan speaks of the liberating effect of embodying this physical amputation, where all the markers of female gender (bar the mouth) are kept in abeyance. Instead, the specular image of the female body is reduced to an entity that barely represents it. On the other hand, Whitelaw writes of the subjective dislocation brought about through this embodiment of incorporating a 'no body':

> If you are blindfolded and have a hood over your face, you hyperventilate, you suffer from sensory deprivation [...] And I hung on and hung

DOI: 10.4324/9781003509622-12

> on until I couldn't any longer. I just went to pieces because I was convinced I was like an astronaut tumbling out into space.
>
> (Billie Whitelaw quoted in Wakeling, [2015], p. 91)

Whitelaw's experience of performing *Not I* gives voice to something fundamental concerning the Beckettian existential landscape in which the presentation of the body is often situated at the intersection of meaning, or the semblance of being and non-being, where nothing of substance, no signifier, no name, can be found to silence the continuous, endless narrations of the psyche. In other words, the physical parameters of the body, as in the case of *Not I, Play* and *The Unnamable*, are substituted by disembodied articulations and the linguistic complexities concerned with interrogating the existence of the personal pronoun 'I'. Alternatively, in less verbally intense monologic performances, such as *Endgame*, a backdrop of silence infiltrates both dialogue and dramatic momentum, and the body is distinctly present in its frailty and contingent inconvenience. Luke Thurston captures this juxtaposition of the body's insistence within derelict, senseless atmospheres in Beckett's drama:

> The disintegration of meaning on the Beckettian stage is always bound up with the body's mute opacity (with what in *Negative Dialectics* (1966) Adorno will call "the somatic, unmeaningful stratum of life" [p. 365], its awkward intrusions onto the terrain of Geist, the 'higher' sphere of the conceptual and semantic.
>
> (Thurston, 2003, p. 35)

While the body may have a senseless dimension, particularly what we can call the Real of the body, the pulsating energy or jouissance of the drives, in *Not I*, we can hardly call it mute, though its visual frame may be absent. It is important to remember that *Not I* falls within the timeframe of the 'later Beckett', a period in which the later plays demonstrate an increasing degree of bodily fragmentation, or a dislocation of voice and body, almost a fading out of the physical body from the parameters of the stage. Ironically, this fading out of the body in *Not I*, along with the incessant speech emanating from a hole in the dark, directly affects the spectators' bodies. In what could be called an Artaudian aesthetic, Beckett said he wanted *Not I* to play on the audience's nerves, thereby bypassing the cognitive avenues of psychic stimulation or rational responses to this piece. It certainly appears to have evoked this disturbing and affect-laden response, as Whitelaw recounts how some audience members tried to run into the toilet to escape the constant stream of language. In this context, theatre is very much the double of life. Given the bodily impact on the nerves of the spectator, *Not I* shows some affinity with the Theatre of Cruelty. Yet, the central dimension of language, spoken words, as a means to provoke the nerves of the spectator, distinguishes it from

Artaud's "affective athleticism" designed to bypass the spoken word, and combined with the minimalist performative style, places *Not I* more in a category of theatre of absence rather than excess. Though, of course, an excess of the body is brought forth through this absence of form, however, the means of provoking it differ from the Theatre of Cruelty—there is a subtraction, a devolving of form rather than an alchemic attempt at transcendence.

There was certainly a cruel dimension to the staging of *Not I*, in terms of how physically and emotionally demanding it was for the actress Billie Whitelaw; she suffered breakdowns and collapsed during one of the rehearsals. Paradoxically, in this play, the absence of the actor's body as a visible image on stage is coupled with the extreme physical discomfort of placing the body in restraints in attempting to act this otherworldly or unearthly role; the body becomes painfully present through the attempt to make it absent. The absence of the physical form juxtaposed with the incessant voice also stages an encounter with the subject of language, or at least the enunciator, as that which is discordant with the body, thus rendering the body more present in its absence. As Anna McMullan argues of Beckett's drama: "The frequent separation of body and voice decentres the subject by creating a position of perception and discourse outside of the body and establishing the body as an object of perception." (2010, p. 10).

Thus, through the absence of the body as an object of perception on the theatrical stage, we, the spectators, view a phenomenon of the everyday in a context that defamiliarises the object by placing it at an altered level of perception. We do not always see clearly the contours of what is most familiar to us and often require an alternate context in which we are 'decentred'. This process of decentring may frame more clearly the particularities of the subject in question.

## Fake Heading 1 – please remove at typesetting stage

### *The Negation of Being*

Despite its novel theatrical form, *Not I* is in keeping with Beckett's previous motifs concerning the existential vagaries of the personal pronoun 'I' and bears a particular affinity with the narrator of *The Unnamable*. However, as scholars have noted, there is an important distinction regarding the momentum and emphasis of this quest, which distinguishes it from the interrogative accent of the latter text. While the narrator in *The Unnamable* meanders down labyrinthine paths of repetitious utterance to perhaps isolate the very singularity of this personal pronoun, *Not I* operates at the level of the shriek, where the narrator is fleeing in a state of terror from this encounter. As Brater puts it, "In *Not I* [...] Mouth is no longer searching for coexistence with its authentic first-person singular, but is instead frantically running away from such an encounter" (Brater, 1974, p. 193). Mouth cannot bear to own her own being, to come face-to-face with the emptiness that is at the core of this being. Of course, it can be argued that we cannot own our own being as it is beyond identification in language but that it is through the very acceptance of its negativity that we come close to it. Llewellyn Brown argues that Mouth's refusal to articulate herself in the first person is a resistance to the language of the Other and hence it is a form of affirmation where she "asserts herself at the level of the drive" and actually comes to be in the very negation of the personal pronoun that would designate her as an ego-subject:

> *She* is the ejaculation that designates the subject as powerless to assume an I, with the result that she comes to being in the energy of this very ejaculation, in this proof of life that, paradoxically, designates her as 'unborn': the subject is situated between the level of the closed utterance (she)—thus resembling the hooded Other—and the abyss where she remains impervious to any naming.
>
> (Brown, 2016, p. 138)

However, what type of being is this that directly corresponds to the drive? Given that the drive is somewhat of a liminal concept, it exists somewhere in between body and mind as a "measure of the demand placed on the mind" to work as a consequence of sensations/feeling/excess in the body. Although the subject of the unconscious cannot be signified concretely as it is not a substantive entity, we can take responsibility for the very elusiveness of the personal pronoun by recognising that where the 'I' leads is to an unnamable source of being. This recognition does not involve a knowing but an acceptance of the unknown, that which can be 'lived but not known'. As Lacan says in *Encore, Seminar XX*, "There is some relationship of being that cannot be known" (1972–1973, p. 119). In effect this means that we cannot know being, at least not in a cognitive sense. I would add that even if knowing being is impossible, we are driven to know something of our being, particularly in states of illness, physical impairment, or limitation, as a means of extending ourselves beyond the unstable parameters of the ego-imaginary self that is in part tied to the body image. When the body comes under strain or recalibrates our being-in-the-world, our very being as subjects often comes into question. Rather than illustrating a direct confrontation with this question, Beckett presents subjects inadvertently driven by a desire to end the discordance of the self—a discordance rendered through the juxtaposition of body and voice, the I and the not-I. Beckett's work appears to be a quest to signify this unnamable, unknowable essence of the subject while always acknowledging its inexpressibility. What signifying this essence implies is debatable but I am inclined to agree with Butler, who takes issue with the idea that Beckett is seeking silence through the endless ramblings of his narrators and places the accent on being:

> Beckett is not seeking silence as such, he is seeking the Being beyond words for which silence is a metaphor or of which it could become an epithet. His continued creation of worlds is a continuing attempt to find the metaphor, the parable, the objective correlative, for Being. A 'nameless' world would be a silent openness to Being and this is what Beckett has been attempting. at least since *The Unnamable.*
>
> (Butler, 1984, p. 179)

If Beckett is seeking being, it is through a process of negation, where the nameless world is exposed in its barren senselessness. In *Not I*, there is a negation of the self or, more precisely, a cancelling of the ego-self and the body that exists as an extension. If "The ego is first and foremost a bodily ego," (Freud, 1923) it is therefore no coincidence that the I and the body are mutually signified by a minus sign (-1). The presentation of the human subject as immobilised and reduced to the restricted corporality of the flesh is a recurring image throughout Beckett's drama and prose. In this play, this motif reaches its apotheosis, and the human subject is collapsed into the representation of one single body part; significantly, the one from which we verbally communicate with the world. I have outlined previously that the body is a source of inherent alienation for the human subject and can be experienced as acutely Other in states of extreme emotional or physical distress. The narrator in *Not I* gives voice to this estrangement within language and the state of being at the mercy of the body. The narrator is helpless in the face of the stream of words emanating from the mouth:

> whole body like gone… just the mouth… lips… cheeks… jaws… never— … what?… tongue?… yes… lips… cheeks… jaws… tongue… never still a second… mouth on fire… stream of words… in her ear… practically in her ear… not catching the half… not the quarter… no idea what she's saying … imagine!… no idea what she's saying!… and can't stop… no stopping it… […] and the whole brain begging… something begging in the brain… begging the mouth to stop.
>
> (Beckett, 1972/2006, p. 380)

We note the pleadings of the narrator, "and the whole brain begging… begging in the brain, begging the mouth to stop". It is not only the body that is partial in *Not I,* but also the sentence structures and the grammatical formulations. The female narrator staggers out, amidst the ellipses, the sentence that the whole body is gone and instead in its place are the individual physical elements comprising the mouth and surrounding facial features (lips, cheeks, jaws). She has been reduced to the terror of the part object of the mouth that refuses to stop, despite the protestations within her brain. Within this torrent of verbal articulations, her experience of the body is cast adrift from the imaginary or narcissistic gestalt of the self (that visual image which provides an illusory but coherent sense of self). As Brater has pointed out, this is an experience where the 'I' is not simply cast adrift but also refused, in a fleeing from the tenuous and unstable normative conditions of bodily coherence.

From its very title, *Not I* alerts us to a negativity, a refusal of ownership, and a statement of denial. As Beckett writes in the directions for the play, "Mouth recovers from vehement refusal to relinquish third person" (Beckett, 1972, p. 375). The narrator in *Not I* refuses to speak in the first person singular, referring to herself as "she", with the cacophony of words and sentences broken into fragments flowing incessantly from the garish orifice. While the fragmented narrative of *Not I* could be said to depict the situation of the poststructuralist subject, unmoored from a central anchor of meaning that would guarantee stability (a subject decentred in relation to the I of the statement), the emphasis is also singular. This particular narrator is not only decentralised but acutely dislocated within her own history and narrative. The woman represented by Mouth is not master of her own thoughts and appears to fade as a subject under the weight of her incessant cognition. Instead of illustrating the Cartesian formulation of "I think therefore I am", Mouth cannot own or accept her individual being as represented by the I statement. In Lacan's reconceptualisation of Descartes's cogito, the being of the subject is foreclosed when the thinking subject is present (as we saw in Chapter 3 regarding alienation). From this perspective, Mouth is fleeing from her being, her words emanating at the speed of thought. In contrast to the conception that this fleeing or negation of being might be symptomatic or pathological, Kyle Gillette, in an article about Zen and the art of self-negation, argues that Mouth's refusal of self illustrates the Zen practice of refuting what we are not and can therefore be aligned with liberation rather than pathology (2012, p. 294). While this is certainly a refreshing perspective, I'm inclined to take the view that Mouth's negation of self is symptomatic in a Lacanian sense, meaning it sheds light on the 'normal' neurotic process of subjecthood as an ongoing stream of thoughts without a definitive anchor of meaning.

### Beyond Pathology

Although it may be tempting to interpret the narrative of this play as the fragmented memory of a particular character who is behind the words, or as a character suffering from a physical illness, and thus provide coherence to the discontinuous stream of consciousness, it is also possible to accept that Beckett has left the character out of the frame in order to present the very lining of what constitutes a body or a self—or to present the self as not whole per se. According to Keir Elam, Beckett's mastery of the art of "leaving out" is achieved in *Not I* in its most spectacular, iconic form, where the very notion of theatrical characterisation is fragmented. Mouth is not a metonym or metaphor for a character (1986, p. 129). In her ephemeral existence, Mouth is literally and metaphorically not all there. As a signifier on the stage, Mouth is an uncanny object, both familiar and strange, alien and intimate. The mouth is the opening to the body's interior, and in this theatrical performance, a dark space that threatens to engulf the spectator with its incessant speech. When we see a human mouth, we expect to see a body, so in *Not I*, something is missing, yet something is omnipotently present within that magnified image.

Through the seductions of interpretation, it may also be tempting to comprehend the jouissance-laden diatribe of *Not I* as a form of psychosis. By making a comparison with Beckett's other works of self-interrogation, in particular that of *The Unnamable*, it is evident that Beckett's art is more a reflection of something universally resonant than the hermetic delusions of an author divorced from 'reality'. As Olga Cox Cameron argues (1994) in an article on *The Unnamable*, the subtleties illustrated by the artistic format concern the aesthetics of a discourse that, while mocking madness, is not madness per se. Beckett's writing, while revealing the mechanisms of a potential experience of psychotic delusion, is not by its nature psychotic, but resonates with all of us to "expose not the silent depths but the ragged clamour at the heart of human subjectivity" (p. 82). Rather than interpreting Mouth's torrent of speech then as psychosis, it can rather serve as a stripped-back image of the body that is already not all there for all subjects.

Similarly, Llewellyn Brown notes that interpretations of *Not I*, like Lois Oppenheim's "normative point of view", which views Mouth "in the light of pathology and impairments" (such as likening Mouth's diatribe to a neurological condition like Tourette Syndrome), paradoxically normalises the alienating and traumatic presence of the voice as jouissance. As he says, "Such an approach ignores jouissance: the question of what inhabits the subject and is at stake for him (2016, p. 122).

In an interpretation and performance of *Not I* by Jess Thom at the Edinburgh Theatre Festival 2017, the fragmented, automated language emanating from a brain that has lost control is given voice through the speech of a woman living with Tourette Syndrome. Mouth's words become punctuated with the ticks and involuntary movements (such as cries of Biscuit) that are part of the condition with which Jess is living. Mouth, therefore, becomes a signifier of a physical condition of the brain, or provides "context" (Gardner, 2017), moving the reception of the performance away from the more indeterminate and psychoanalytically symptomatic resonances of the original text. This interpretation of Beckett's monologue aligns with the current and growing research on reading for disability in his work as a whole, which I have discussed in Chapter 4 in light of his fantasy of debility.

It is interesting that situating Mouth within the light of a physical impairment is categorised as a "normative point of view", given that physical difference is often considered non-normative. However, this is where the subtlety of Beckett's representation of the body comes to the fore, as to consider Mouth within the light of a medical condition might be to miss the inherently alienating and traumatic immanent processes of the body as they occur for everyone, including what Lacan in later years referred to as the parasitic dimension of language. Language is Other to the body, colonising it with words and meaning we have not invented. From this perspective, speech is a foreign agent that invades the subject, capable of "inflicting suffering comparable to an illness" (Brown, 2016, p. 243). In *Seminar XXIV*, Lacan literally tied the notion of the body to the signifier as operating partly in the Real and interestingly in the dark:

> There is, for this knot, a cord. The cord is also *corps-de* (body-of). This *corps-de*, is parasited on by the signifier; for the signifier though it forms part of the Real, it is indeed there that I am right to situate the Symbolic, one must think of the following, which is that we might well have dealings with this *corps-de* only in the dark.
>
> (Lacan, Lesson 7, 15 February 1977, p. 88)

In this passage, Lacan is equivocal with the word cord and draws a connection between the idea of a knot and the body. The body is the body of (*corps-de*) the signifier; it is knotted as would be a cord. In this sense, language invades the body as a parasite or a vine ensnared within the body's very organism. Of course, it is also possible to incorporate both these viewpoints (that of disability and that of the jouissance of the signifier) in an appraisal of the resonances of Mouth's alienating rendition. That is to say, one can be subject to the vagaries and impositions of a medical condition at the same time as being subject to the jouissance that pervades all human beings to some degree or another—indeed, they bear an interesting relationship.

As we have seen in previous chapters, the human body, as we are conceiving it, is not a whole entity in the sense of being unified and complete, a thing in itself, but is rather a body that has holes or indeed a body that, as Jacques-Alain Miller (2019) puts it, is in pieces. These holes relate to the inability of the signifier to fully drain the jouissance of the flesh and the impossibility of ever obtaining full knowledge or reaching a final signified for the experience of the body. Holes, of course, also relate to the orifices of the body that are like attractor basins for enjoyment, such as the mouth, the anus, the vagina, the ear. If the body is composed of holes, what is the being of the body in this sense? In *Encore*, Lacan explicitly says that if there is something that grounds being, it is the body (1972–1973, p. 110). However, we have seen that the term body does not indicate which aspect of the body or register it refers to, so this statement is a little confusing, given the subject's discordance with the body. Furthermore, in the same seminar, he refers specifically to the "being of the body" as that of the sexed being (p. 5). Here, Lacan appears to be distinguishing between the sexed body and the living body. However, it may be that there is a vacillation in his thinking concerning the body and being. He repeats something that he says at various stages in his seminars: the unknowability of the living body:

> The substance of the body, on the condition that it is defined only as that which enjoys itself (*se jouit*). That is, no doubt, a property of the living body, but we don't know what it means to be alive except for the following fact, that a body is something that enjoys itself (*cela se jouit*).
> (1972–1973, p. 23)

What does it mean to say the body enjoys itself? Lacan indicates that jouissance lies in simply having a body or in simply being alive, and that we are not in cognitive control over how we enjoy, even though we may give rationalisations for why we do things. To put it simply, there is an excess —a drive to release or use energy operating within the body—but we can never completely drain it away as long as we are alive. In essence, I am equating the jouissance of the body with a form of energy, affectual excitation, or satisfaction at the level of the flesh.[1] We can also think of the autoerotic[2] act of masturbation as a way that the body has of enjoying itself and obtaining release or pleasure from heightened excitation by inducing excitation. As Alexandre Stevens (2021) puts it:

> This jouissance of the body is not simply that of a body insofar as it enjoys, but of a body insofar as it enjoys of itself. This is not at all the same thing, since this body that enjoys of itself is thus the body of autoeroticism. This is the real of the body in the last Lacan.

By autoeroticism, we can think of the concept of One that Lacan invokes in various ways, from the unary trait to the One all alone. We enjoy through an Other but also as something unique to ourselves. Only we can feel our desire for the Other or the anxiety that accompanies desire, as the potential loss of the esteemed object shadows our enjoyment. A certain enjoyment or jouissance of the body is not divisible by the lack-inducing properties of the signifier. As part object, Mouth is both the absence of a body and the body writ large as the subject of the drive. We literally have a figure for the acephelous subject that enjoys as if it were an other. There is no relation to the other as in a typical fantasy of two seemingly intact subjects who enjoy each other or need each other to ratify their existence. There is no such thing as the sexual relation (Lacan, 1972–1973), meaning we engage with the object of our fantasy (as enjoyment) through the being of the other, but we do not directly relate to the other.

### ***Mouth As Erogenous Zone***

To argue that *Not I* is a dramatic work that illustrates the sexual non-rapport might seem far-fetched. What could be remotely sexual about an isolated mouth ranting and raving in the dark, with nothing but language echoing in this empty space? Yet, it is precisely this isolation of the mouth as part object of the body that represents an erogenous zone where pleasure and jouissance converge. Mouth's suspension in the dark delimits what Lacan calls an erogenous zone of the body with its discreet components of lips, teeth, tongue: "At the erogenous level we speak of the mouth, of the lips and the teeth, of what Homer calls the enclosure of the teeth" (1964/1978, p. 169).

In psychoanalytic terms, the mouth is the orifice corresponding to the oral drive, one of the constituents in the series of partial drives schematised by Lacan as anal, scopic, oral, and invocatory.[3] The drives relate to the holes in the body around which pleasure and a relationship to others converge, such as the eyes, anus, and mouth. The mouth is not only an erogenous zone stimulated through sexual activity but is also the organ implicated in the act of speech and language. We speak words with our mouths and perform a transformation of thought to signification. In Lacanian terms, the voice is one of the 'objects' relating to the invocatory drive and is a cause of subjective desire. As a sound, it originates within the body, yet it can appear to be cut off from this body, manifesting as the uncanny, something that is alien or strange and yet familiar. In states of psychosis, voices that appear to originate from the outside world and which form a persecutory and invasive presence can be disavowed voices of the internal psyche. This phenomenon underlines the significance of the voice as an object that can exist as an experience of something alien, a presence that can be traumatic and perceived as intrusive by the psyche.

According to Lacan, the voice resonates in the body as it corresponds with the orifice of the ear, which, in contrast to the other orifices, cannot be shut. (Lacan, 1964, p. 195). The orifices of the body are sites of potential pleasure, either through the fulfilment of need and sexual satisfaction and consequently are also potential sites of jouissance. Where there is pleasure for the human subject, there is also the potential for excess, an excess that often enjoys at our expense. The spectacle of Mouth performs this paradox of the human subject's relationship to enjoyment and the partial drives, as something intrinsic and yet alien to the self. This type of enjoyment is not simply performed through the act of sex, but as part of the very symbolic structures that make up our everyday world. Lacan proposed that language is a form of jouissance at the level of speech and therefore that sexuality and its concomitant 'enjoyment' is not just attributable to sexual acts but is enveloped within the very act of speaking. In other words, there is an enjoyment in and of the signifier. The very act of speaking is a mode of enjoyment, a means of jouissance for the one who speaks. As Lacan puts it: "For the moment, I am not fucking, I am talking to you. Well! I can have exactly the same satisfaction as if I were fucking" (1964, p. 165).

Therefore, if satisfaction is inherent to speech, we can conceive of the jouissance of the signifier as something that lies between meaning (as it concerns the Other) and the organism of the body, as that which is unknowable in a cognitive sense. It is neither solely natural, as in a pregiven fact of physical existence, nor is it purely in the realm of culture, as something that inhabits us from without.

In *Not I*, Mouth functions as a synecdoche of the body and provides an image of a form that signifies the paradox of pleasure and jouissance attributable to this orifice. As an autonomous and singular agent of the performance, Mouth is animated without being animate, an object without an owner. This acephalous narrator denies the enjoyment of her own experiences and does not position herself in the place of I (as the enunciator of the statement). Instead, language as a corollary to the enjoying substance of the body enjoys in the place of the I. Indeed, Mouth captures this displacement of enjoyment in her denial of the first-person pronoun. It is not *I* who is enjoying but *she*. The narrator expresses a time that might have been related to a sexual experience where she did not feel pleasure:

> just as the odd time... in her life... when clearly intended to be having pleasure ... she was in fact... having none... not the slightest
>
> (Beckett, 1972/2006, p. 377)

Although professing that she did not experience pleasure, paradoxically, the expression of this experience in *Not I* indicates a jouissance at the level of speaking. The human mouth is a vehicle for pleasure in acts of eating, drinking, speaking, and sexuality, but all these activities also contain a possibility for jouissance, a going beyond the pleasure principle and a drive toward death. It is precisely because no object of any kind can satisfy the drive that the mouth as oral orifice corresponding to the drive is insatiable. As Lacan states: "Even when you stuff the mouth—the mouth that opens in the register of the drive—it is not the food that satisfies it, it is as one says, the pleasure of the mouth" (Lacan, 1964/1978, p. 67). Therefore, we can obtain pleasure through the very act of putting something in the mouth and not simply from the object that we may be eating. The pleasure of the mouth need not have a teleological purpose, such as the satiation of need or the feeling of hunger.

As is characteristic of references to sexuality and sexual organs in Beckett's work, there is an ambivalence inherent to this presentation of Mouth; it is both an object of erotic lure and an object of disgust.[4] Appearing as an orifice that is spitting and raving, it is also symbolic of the female sex organ. Indeed Mouth, as it spews forth words, is redolent of an evacuation orifice, and given Beckett's conflation between the vagina and the anus in Molloy (the anus as the birth canal), Mouth becomes an image suggestive of all of these orifices. This particular magnification of lips, teeth and tongue is also resonant in its specular form of the vagina (Elam, 1986). Similarly, Freud had observed the symbolism of the mouth in *The Interpretation of Dreams* and wrote that the image of a mouth and other part objects of the body in a dream may be symbolic and representative of the genitals: "The genitals may even be represented in dreams by other parts of the body: the male member by the hand or the foot, the female genital orifice by the mouth, the ear, or even the eye". (Freud, 1900, p. 171). In *The Three Essays on Sexuality*, Freud notes the non-totalising component of the sexual drive and its tendency to become aligned with individual parts of the body. Therefore, existing as a part object on the border of the erotic and the alien, the erogenous and the abject, Mouth captures the polymorphous perversity of sexuality beneath the imaginary gestalt of wholeness (where two become one), perpetuated by popular culture.

The depiction of sexual part objects is a frequent occurrence in Beckett's work, and references to sexuality and sexual acts are often mechanistic and empirical, devoid of pleasure and eroticism. The needs and eroticisations of the body are represented with an almost animalistic quality where the sexual acts are hinged on instinct (as a compulsion) and not from desire. In some respects, Beckett's depictions of sexuality, reproduction and love resonate with what has become formulated in contemporary times as an anti-relational queer perspective.[5] Sexuality is 'enjoyed' without the end goal of reproduction, and where the connection between sex and death is laid bare. In keeping with this view, with his depictions of truncated selves, Beckett refuses the fantasy of Oneness that veils the trauma of the absence of the sexual relation. *In Not I*, the satisfaction of the drive is conveyed through the image of a truncated body, and a brain that goes on buzzing, tormented by an insatiable impulse to speak. In Lacanian terms, the drive is always partial and associated with the different orifices and libidinal intensities of the body; it obtains satisfaction in a piecemeal fashion, but can never be fully satisfied. It circulates around the object as satisfaction rather than through its absence as desire. In this sense, the Mouth in *Not I* is not simply presenting the object a as an absence but also as an excessive presence. The relation to the Other, however, is still indicated as a lack, a barred Other. This is because, despite the fragmented stream of words and the specular image of a part body, rather than a whole character, the drama of *Not I* is nonetheless structured around a semblance of sender-receiver communication. That is to say that despite this spectacle of ultimate subjective alienation, from self and other, the Other as receiver of the communication is present in some fashion: "Although Mouth speaks, Auditor hears, and audience sees" (Brater, 1987, p. 19). The auditor is a hooded, indeterminate figure and can only respond helplessly to Mouth with vague gestures indicating her inability to aid her distress. In this way, he or she serves a purpose as a semblance of the vaguest possibility of communication, a silent but significant receptacle of the female narration. The presence of the auditor tempers the solipsism of the performance and suggests that in order to exist as a subject, there must always be someone to whom we address our speech. *Not I* illustrates the presence of the Other as a structuring principle through which the relation to the object a as a fantasy of debility is present via symbolic representations of absence and organs without bodies. *In Not I*, the object a is both present as an absence and a disturbing excess—a discord in the field of the visible.

The play's performative dimension is disturbing at the level of identification with the body as an imaginary Gestalt. The spectator of *Not I* is not permitted the fantasy of relation through a 'whole' body that could shield us from entering the hole-body or the abyss of Mouth's fragmented world. The darkness of the stage setting defines the physical outlines of Mouth and delimits a hole in the body that is suspended in space rather than attached to a physical form. The physicality of Mouth speaks to the corporeal substance of the human subject, while also serving as a metaphor for the substanceless void interior to subjectivity. Thus, the amputated part object of Mouth contextualises the human subject as disembodied, fragmented and deterritorialised. Within this alienating spectacle, the gaze (that which actively directs our look) of the spectator is dislocated from the normative strictures of habitual perception. In other words, we have no imaginary gestalt with which to identify; the contours of identification are deformed or disturbed through this confrontation with a hole that somehow draws us into its interior by speaking so fast we relate to the inner torment of the I voice. Something of the being of the subject in its subjection to language is externalised and the discord with the body is also represented by the cloaking of the framing darkness. The gaze of the spectator is subverted through the sensory deprivation of the performance, and instead of being seduced by a spectacle that presents the ego (through the illusion of a whole character) as an autonomous agent, the audience encounters the reality of the enjoying body, a confrontation with tormenting jouissance. Similar to *Endgame*, there is no presence of anything normative that could set up a contrast between an ideal body and a debilitated one. Instead there is an absence where a body should be, perhaps the ultimate representation of the unknowable/intangible aspect of the trauma of the body. The absence marks the divide between the being of the subject and the being of the body. Mouth is situated on the border—a rim marking the hole encapsulated by the body. As we saw in Chapter 3, according to Lacan's perspective on alienation in *Seminar XI*, the being of the subject is not to be experienced through words and meaning; rather, a bifurcation occurs between being and meaning, or between body and subject. In order to speak, to take up a position in language, there is something of our being that we give up or that is effaced in the process of acceding to the status of a speaking being. However, there is somewhat of a slippage here between the body and being, as a pound of flesh (in Lacan's words) has been given up to enter into the symbolic—so something of being and something of the body would seem to be missing. Or even something of being as it relates to the body, is missing. While this aspect is missing, it is still what we are. However, we may not be able to speak it, causing a certain repetition or rhythmic intensity of affect encircling around this absent cause, just like Mouth's insistent diatribe.

This slippage between being and having a body is illustrated in Beckett's pared-back world, where language oscillates in the gaps opened by the body's inherent instability. On the one hand, the body seems to be the *sine qua non* of the lack endemic to the human subject, emphasised by its imperfection and limitations, a grounding of being in the humility of the 'I do not know'; on the other, Beckett attempts to transcend its biological impositions through the elevating of words as the path to find a final signifier that would bring silence to the mind's endless locubrations. In his staging of the bifurcation of language and the body, we are more than the shit and mud of our material existence through which we drag ourselves and being is tied to an absence that cannot be said but which drives the urge to speak. Mouth depicts the Cartesian aspect of Beckett's drama, where the mind keeps on talking and raving, despite the lack of a body, thus demonstrating the impossible scenario of a human being living as an organ without a body or as a speaking subject disconnected from the materiality of the body. There is a certain ambivalence about the materiality of the body in Beckett's drama; it is both a pathway to the truth of being and an obstacle that Beckett might like to remove altogether.

## Notes

1 This perspective on jouissance is very debatable and there is no specific consensus about what exactly the 'substance' of jouissance constitutes. Personally I think that if there is an economy of jouissance, phallic, body, etc., we have to be dealing with different qualities of affect. In borrowing a turn of phrase from Mark Solms, jouissance must surely 'feel' like something.

2 Darian Leader (2021) makes the point that autoeroticism also involves the Other, thereby complications notions of jouissance that foreclose the Other.

3 In *The Book of Love and Pain* (2004), Nasio argues that pain is also an object of the drive.

4 Molloy: "Unfortunately it is not of them I have to speak, but of her who brought me into the world, through the hole in her arse if my memory is correct. First taste of the shit" (Beckett, 1958, p. 12).

5 For example, as explored in the work of Lee Edelman (2004), *Queer Theory and the Death Drive.* For Edelman, the figure of the queer, as situated in a non-teleological sexuality is the ultimate embodiment of the death drive.

## References


Beckett, S. (1972). Not I. In *Samuel Beckett. The complete dramatic works* (pp. 373–385): Croydon: Faber & Faber.

Brator, E. (1974). The "I" in Beckett's *Not I*. *Twentieth-Century Literature*, 20 (4), 189–200.

Brown, L. (2016). *Beckett, Lacan and the voice*. Ibidem.

Butler, L. S. J. (1984). *Samuel Beckett and the meaning of being: A study in ontological parable*. Macmillan.

Cox Beckett, O. (1994). Beckett's Unnamable: Not I, not mad. *The Letter*, (1), 82–94.

Elam, K. (1986). Not I: Beckett's mouth and the ars(e) rhetotica. In E. Brater, *Beckett at 80/Beckett in context* (pp. 124–148). New York: Oxford University Press.

Freud, S. (1900). *The interpretation of dreams*. Retrieved from www.abika.com.

Gardner, L. (2017). Not I review – Jess Thom gives Beckett's motor mouth extra bite. *The Guardian*, 27 August. Retrieved 27 October 2019.

Gillette, Kyle (2012) Zen and the art of self-negation in Samuel Beckett's *Not I*. *Comparative Drama*. 46 (3), Article 2.

Lacan, J. (1964/1978). *The seminar of Jacques Lacan. Book XI. The Four Fundamental Concepts of Psychoanalysis*. (J.-A. Miller, ed., & A. Sheridan, transl.) New York: Norton.

Lacan, J. (1972–1973/1999). *Encore. Book XX. On feminine sexuality and the limits of love and knowledge*. (J.-A. Miller, ed., & B. Fink, transl.) New York: Norton.

Lacan, J. (1976–1977). *L'insu que sait … Seminar XXIV Final Sessions 1–12*. (C. Gallagher, transl.) Unpublished.

McMullan, A. (2010). *Theatre on trial: Samuel Beckett's later drama*. Routledge.

Miller, J.-A. (2019). *Lacanian biology and the event of the body, part II*. Lacan.com.

Stevens, A. (2021). The body marked by language. *Νέα Λακανική Σχολή Ψυχαναλυσης*. Webpage.

Thurston, L. (2003). Meaning on trial: Sublimation and the reader. In P. Adams (Ed), *Art sublimation or symptom* (pp. 29–49). Karnac.

Wakeling, C. (2015). "Only her mouth could move": Sensory deprivation and the Billie Whitelaw plays. *Drama Review*, 59 (3) 91–107.

Chapter 9

# After Artaud

## The Body as the Question of Being

Bodies that scream, limbs falling from the sky, vivid descriptions of physical and emotional pain, invocations of affect and jouissance: Artaud's writings and theatrical work depict a body subject to the trauma of language and the cruel contingencies of life. While Beckett's work is more closely associated with disability theories, Artaud's quest to reformulate being through the deformations of the body provides additional scope for thinking about disability or the critique of ableism. Furthermore, from the perspective of the body as a somatopsychic phenomenon, Artaud's emphasis on the matter of the body, his attempts to invent a new body through the body without organs, and its potential influence on disability studies, although featured in the field, appear yet to reach fruition. It is worthwhile asking why someone so focused on the lived experience of the body, its pains, jouissance and torments, as is Artaud, is not considered very notable within these fields. It is clear that his work poses a resistance to ableism and to normative, idealistic conceptions of the mind–body relation, both in the bringing forth of the sufferings of the physical body and in the area of mental health, as Artaud is strongly associated with the anti-psychiatry movement. His work and writings contain concrete protests against electroshock treatment and his general confinement in the asylums of his later life. As Artaud's dramatic work, particularly his staged work, is limited, this chapter will not be an analysis of a specific play but will identify the performative dimension of Artaud's concept of the body-without-organs within contemporary culture and how it can provide insight into Artaud's evolution of attempting to ground being through the body. Is there something about being and its relation to the body within the context of disability that remains to be said, in the sense that it cannot be said but insists within the experience of having a body, maybe even more so in states of physical illness, psychic distress, and non-normative embodiment? What is the relation between being and the body?

As I have postulated, from a Lacanian perspective, being is not a monistic concept but is fragmented, discordant, and non-unitary. It is not simply that the subject is divided between the conscious and the unconscious, the ego and the id but is divided in its very being, as a subject of the signifier and a subject of

DOI: 10.4324/9781003509622-13

jouissance (a jouissance of the Real of the body), though of course, to complicate this, the signifier is also a source of jouissance. I reiterate that the signifier in a Lacanian sense, although it is often equated with language, is not simply words or language in the linguistic form but is anything that signals or induces meaning effects. Importantly, division does not imply a binary or an either/or but a segmentation or breaking up, a separation into parts. It can be tempting to be seduced by the idea of two distinct parts, yet with human subjectivity, we are not dealing with something so 'clear cut' or measurable empirically. Fundamentally, the truth of being concerns or overlaps with the question of what is life—what constitutes the spark of our existence or the nature of life in its essential form—or tangentially, as I have been asking in this book: what is the body? As discussed in a 2025 ICLO cartel presentation, the question of life still remains unanswered definitively. In the words of Jacques-Alain Miller (2010), this question is intimately bound with that of the body:

> We do not know what life is. We only know that there is no *jouissance* without life. And why not formulate the principle in this way: life is the condition of *jouissance*. But that is not all. It is precisely a matter of life under the form of the body. *Jouissance* is unthinkable without the living body, itself the condition of *jouissance*.

While being is a massively complex philosophical phenomenon, a full discussion of which is beyond the remit of this book, I refer to it as signifying the background properties of existence per se, what defines our particular manifestation as singular yet interrelated subjects, and what constitutes the presence or affective dimension of our bodies. In many aspects, and Lacan says this in *Encore* (1972–1973), the body is the ground of being, as without a body, we would not exist, at least not in our current form. However, with the rise of AI, posthumanism is alive and well, and the question is now pressing whether we, or machinic entities, can exist as consciousness without a human body or how extensions of our bodies through technological apparatuses and prosthetics constitute us as biologically human. In our digitally mediated times, the materiality of the body is increasingly under erasure, either through the reduction of jobs that can now be done by machines or through the nature of social communication through devices, social media, and video calls. As a result, the nature of being and the constituents of life are changing, or at least being contested. We may be entering the era of bodies without organs, bodies that speak of a machinic transformation of being through the invention of a new body—a body not restricted by the physical organism. This poses exciting possibilities for those with disabilities but also some alarming potentialities for human relationality and ethical issues surrounding artificial consciousness.

While now a famous philosophical term, Artaud used the term 'the body without organs' only once in his 1948 radio production, *To Have Done with the Judgment of God*. It was the work of Gilles Deleuze and Félix Guattari that reified this concept as a figure of the immortal, an inspiration for thinkers grappling with the limits of the body in attempts to transcend normative conceptions of embodiment, such as those pertinent to ableism. This phrase or concept, including the timeframe of its emergence, marks an apotheosis of Artaud's life's work and legacy. It marks a shift from the earlier Artaud of the Theatre of Cruelty in the 1930s to the late Artaud, or what has been referred to as the post-Rodez Artaud, of the mid to late 1940s. Artaud's theatrical work did not stop with nor is confined to a reading of plays within his repertoire of the Theatre of Cruelty; it could be argued that his own body becomes the site of an attempt at corporeal transformation, a performance through a composition of screams and cries and glossolalia, of a body disintegrated and fragmentated, yet paradoxically resurrected from the torture of electroshock treatment, addiction and psychosis. In his later years, Artaud's inventiveness in finding solutions to the trauma of the body as an existential phenomenon and to the trauma of *his* body as a singular encounter shone through the fragmentary, undead characters of his drawings and in the creation of an impossible body: the body without organs.

## The Cultural Impact of the Body Without Organs

> When you will have made him a body without organs,
> then you will have delivered him from all his automatic reactions
> and restored him to his true freedom.
> They you will teach him again to dance wrong side out
> as in the frenzy of dance halls
> and this wrong side out will be his real place.
>
> (Artaud, 1947)

In his 1947 radio piece *To Have Done with the Judgment of God*, Artaud's post-Rodez artistic work reaches or surpasses the limits of the intelligible. A strange and eerie performance of glossolalia, shrieks, screams, and incantatory music, the piece was shelved the day before it was due to be broadcast. Artaud died a month later. It is poignant that, just before his death, Artaud would speak of the invention of a new body, which, in my understanding, would not be limited by the organic dimension of the human body, a dimension, as we have seen, that is never purely material but also discursive. What could an organ-less body be and why is it such a seductive concept? On the one hand, it seems that a body that lacks organs, the very substance that gives it life, cannot be a living body, in the sense that we have identified it, a body which suffers or enjoys jouissance. It must be an imaginary construct, an image of a body that is not whole in the typical sense of corporeal integration, but formulated or whole in such a way as to provide a freedom from the very dissonance that the realm of the imaginary produces in us. It is what

Brenner (2021), in his work on the autistic body, refers to as a "body without holes", given that organs obtain significance from the structuring and traumatic effects of language on the body. Our organs are fleshy entities that sustain life but they also exist at the level of signification and metaphor—a 'broken heart', 'no leg to stand on', 'my heart in my mouth', etc. While a shattering of the body without 'organs' situates the body in a state of disorganisation or destratification, as Deleuze and Guattari put it, that is outside the 'organs' of meaning, a disassemblage of the body may also be an attempt at a unification of body and mind through the breaking up of a body that is problematic, traumatic and codified by convention. In this way, fragmentation becomes defragmentation, a way of processing, reorganising, and, indeed, re-codifying the inherent disorder constitutive of embodiment and subjectivity. The body without organs is a paradox, implying a negation 'without' that creates an entity which lacks lack, therefore a body that is somewhat complete or empty of the signifier and yet only exists as a function of the signifier. In other words, it has no substantial essence. As Deleuze and Guattari put it, "You never reach the Body without Organs, you can't reach it, you are forever attaining it, it is a limit" (1987, p.105).

Artaud's invention of this concept, and its wide appeal as a concept or, at the very least, a turn of phrase in academic circles, including its reversal to organs without bodies (Žižek, 2004), points to a collective desire to extend the parameters of subjectivity by redefining or interrogating what we know to be the limits of the body. It highlights how the body is a continuous question of discourse, indeed how the concept of it functions as a product of discourse, let alone a question for individual subjects. Of course, for Artaud, it also signals the emergence of what Jay Murphy (2016) refers to as his singularity, in particular as it relates to his later works, which, as Murphy notes, despite experiencing the horrors of his psychiatric confinement and the ravages of electric shock treatment, dwarf the output of his earlier period. Artaud's drawings and art from his later period illustrate both the fragmentation and construction of an alternate body. One of his drawings is entitled "The True Body" indicating the falsity and discordance of the original one. The body without organs is the apotheosis of Artaud's corporeal project: a means of accessing and reconfiguring being through the body. What does this mean? Fundamentally, there is something that is out of sync or which, at the level of the drives, causes a disruption at the imaginary level between being and having. Artaud does not simply *have* a body; he *is* his body and wants to convey this through his writings. Because he is his body, and the body is a torment, he wants to radically alter it and, by so doing, reorganise the grounds of being. Although Lacan says in *Seminar XXIII, Joyce and the Sinthome* (1975–1976), that we are essentially not a body but have one, I think we can find vacillations in his conceptions of being as aligned with the body, as we have seen, for example, in *Seminar XX, Encore*, but also moments where the body is distinctly not in accord with the unconscious and hence with being. There is a view in psychoanalysis that we are identified with the body image but are not the body. As Miller (2010) puts it, "Psychoanalysis makes its space in the lack of this identification between being and body, in maintaining that the subject has a relationship of having with the body." That being said, I think there is also space for psychoanalysis to consider the ramifications of the subject also being the body, at least in part. While this presupposes complex questions about the nature of the subject of the unconscious and its arguable nonsubstantiality, my point is that there is something about the organic body that influences this subject in ways currently undeterminable. Perhaps the subject vacillates between the being of the unconscious as the signifier and the being of the body as jouissance, as being subject to jouissance, but neither complements the other as two parts of a whole.

While we can speculate on the clinical context of this insight, in Artaud's case, the consequence of psychosis and a deficit at the level of the imaginary, for example—perhaps the imaginary body, borne of the identification with the body image at the mirror stage, does not function well for Artaud—I would rather, for the most part, stay with the universal resonances of this insistence of corporeal being, in particular how it relates to states of disability, pain and suffering. However, I will venture first with a singular explanation in Artaud's case. We must consider the complexity of jouissance as it arises in Lacan's thought and how it relates to being. If the human subject is divided in its very being, then we are divided between the jouissance of the body as a living entity and that of the signifier. While the jouissance of the symbolic is referred to in Lacanian terms as phallic jouissance, an enjoyment I understand to be related to the desire of the Other and the satisfactions of obtaining recognitions, status and identification in the face of this Other, the jouissance of the Real of the body, this being of the body, is more archaic, meaningless, and unfiltered by signification. Although we are dealing with different modalities of jouissance and I would infer different qualitative affects, it would be a mistake to treat them as distinctly separate or as if they could be neatly categorised in a hierarchical economy. Mari Ruti captures this when she describes how the signifier cannot fully dismember the real and empty it of jouissance. There is always something of the original jouissance present:

> The remaining traces, scraps, residues, or leftovers of jouissance continue to destabilize the subject, threatening to dismantle it from within even as they simultaneously animate and support its embodied existence. This, I would concede, is an existential 'crisis' of potentially formidable proportions.
>
> (2012, p. 20)

Although an existential dilemma for all subjects, the management of jouissance is impacted by singular traumatic events and clinical structure. The body without organs was a way for Artaud to deal with the invasion of jouissance as the Real of the body, a Real that for him was disordered in such a way that the very organs of the body were oppressively present. The body was both a site of suffering, a reminder that being has a material quality, and a portal for transcendence in its demolition. As Murphy (2015) writes: "Through it [the body without organs] Artaud intends to abolish interiority once and for all and forgo the limitations of the physical flesh" (paragraph 3). On which register does the body without organs function? Is it a deformation of the imaginary, something which can alter the subject at the level of identification, or is it another image or identification which ultimately shields the subject from the incoherence of being, albeit an image of fragmentation (*without* organs), or is it something that operates on the Real, a way of actually reorganising subjectivity? Perhaps it operates across all three registers as a concept that knots the imaginary and the Real. In other words, there is potential to view it as what Lacan calls a sinthome—a way of holding the body together through the construction of a new imaginary element that functions to provide substance to the Real. Even if the body without organs is an imaginary construct—it is composed of words and constitutes an image—its driving force is the desire to bypass the limiting stratifications of the symbolic, the divisionary and traumatic impact of language on the demarcation of the organs of the body, what Deleuze and Guattari refer to as the organisation of the organism.

> We come to the gradual realization that the BwO is not at all the opposite of the organs. The organs are not its enemies. The enemy is the organism. The BwO is opposed not to the organs but to that organization of the organs called the organism. It is true that Artaud wages a struggle against the organs, but at the same time what he is going after, what he has it in for, is the organism: *The body is the body. Alone it stands. And in no need of organs.*
>
> (1987, p. 158)

This potential to re-envisage the construction of the organism reveals the importance of the body without organs in contemporary scholarship. In an essay on how the body without organs envisages an autistic relationship to the body as a way of bypassing the symbolic, Leon Brenner (2021) advocates for a clinical appraisal of this concept by applying Deleuze and Guattari's reading of Artaud's concept in *A Thousand Plateaus* to develop current Lacanian understandings both of autism and the body. He writes that for Deleuze and Guattari, the body without organs of the masochistic and schizophrenic subject is a body that succeeds in annulling the Other. Yet their account is based on a misreading of Lacan's registers of psychosis and perversion. It is in fact the autistic subject who provides the clinical support for their concept (p. 47). For the autistic subject, who has what Brenner calls "an empty body without organs" (p. 47), due to the absence of the symbolic ordering of the body, jouissance can invade and disturb without the mitigation of castration. However, the "full autistic body without organs" (p. 49), which involves the use of objects as adjuncts for the body, allows for a conceptualisation of the singularity of being for the autistic subject that does not pathologise or attempt to normalise the less symbolically mediated relation to the body.

The body without organs provides a path to consider other avenues of non-normative embodiment. In her work on a post-structuralist, post-humanist approach to disability, Shildrick utilises a Deleuzian account of the body without organs to envisage a pathway of becoming in which the disabled body has greater possibilities for valuation than other paradigms of embodiment. She argues: "the significance of Deleuzian notions like 'desiring machine', 'assemblage', and 'body without organs' [are] all terms that have the potential to radically disrupt the devaluation of the disabled body" (2009, p. 125). From this perspective, the disabled body is not limited to the actual physical dimensions of the flesh; it can be transformed through the metaphorisation of its potential within a system of relating fundamentally associated with its phenomenal actuality. A simple example could be the different ways in which having certain knowledge of the body's vulnerability can play out, or the interactions with people that occur as a consequence of the disability. There are many valuable aspects of having a disability or impairment that are not accounted for by standard ableist notions of what constitutes a desirable body or existence, not least as can be the case for many people that the disability, due for instance to an incapacity to work in a typical sense, slows a person down and brings about a more reflective, less materialistic-neoliberal focused state of being. However, I think there is potential, though, with theories of becoming and rhizomatic systems of revaluation, to overlook states of extreme suffering within categories of disability that simply resist having any intrinsic value or sense whatsoever. Perhaps an antidote to this utopia of becoming is an application of the body without organs from the perspective of Artaud's engagement with being, undiluted by Deleuze and Guattari's interpretation. Of course, this poses the problem of signification, as we cannot fully interpret the 'meaning' of the body without organs for Artaud, not least as it is a construct that takes issue with meaning per se but also as it may indeed have been an enigma for him too. One of the most comprehensive accounts of Artaud's concept within the context of his oeuvre has to be that given by Jay Murphy in *Artaud's Metamorphosis: From Hieroglyphs to Bodies without Organs*, where Murphy traces the origins of this 'new body' in Artaud's involvement with the rites and rituals of the Tarahumara Indians in Mexico, through to his transformation after his incarcerations in mental institutions. Murphy captures the nuances of Artaud's battle with signification and the body over time, and does not succumb to generalisations of Artaud's work that define his position towards language as something static but rather evolving. We can trace the body without organs then as something evolving through Artaud's theatrical experiments or inventions, not simply in the theatre within the productions of staged plays, but as performative within his last radio production. It is both a concept, a signifier composed of words, but also a bodily event evident in the decomposition of language in *To Have Done with the Judgment of God*. The shrieks, cries and glossolalia are a means for Artaud to access what Lacan calls lalangue, the raw, undifferentiated jouissance-laden underbelly of language that has a particular corporeal dimension. As Bernard Pocheret puts it, lalangue is:

> the material consisting of sounds, phonemes and words in their raw state and not articulated into the structure of a discourse—material that collides with living bodies. Lalangue is something that is endured or suffered. It is a passion. Human beings are the patients of this encounter between lalangue and the body.

We can also remember that the scream is the ultimate signifier of a body in pain, and the earliest sign of a baby's distress to its caregiver—a signifier of helplessness and powerlessness or the inherent vulnerability of the self. Tubino and Moschen (2021) consider the place of the scream in Artaud's work as a bridge to the unutterable and note that, although Artaud was unaware of Lacan's neologism, lalangue, some of it was transmitted through his work (p. 3).

Perhaps the body without organs is the conceptual index of a body that suffers from lalangue; it is an attempt at liberation through the invention of a new body that does not conform to the limitations of signification but an acknowledgement of the suffering at the heart of the body's enjoying substance. It provides access to the being of the body as the jouissance of the Real of the body—that aspect we cannot speak of but perhaps can still give voice to. I had said that in Artaud's case, he did not simply *have* a relation to his body but *was* his body in the sense of being. However, I think we can extend it to all subjects with the caveat that there are variations in clinical structure and singularity; how can we say that our identification with the signifier is not somehow corporeal to begin with, the spark of our very existence as subjects, and that, therefore, the imaginary has binding effects at the level of being, not simply at the level of the ego? Or indeed that the ego itself has its roots in being. I mentioned at the beginning of this book that the ego has a very close relationship with the body, as seen in states of illness, pain, and disability. There can be a literal resurrection or a deflation of the ego, depending on the level of energy in the body. The imaginary, then, is also tied to the Real of the body, to the drives that pulsate and clamour for release—it is a means of regulating them. What happens when there is narcissistic injury or when the ego comes under attack from forces internal to the body, as in pain, excessive sensation, overwhelming jouissance or indeed from forces external in the social realm, such as ostracisation, marginalisation and lack of recognition? If the thread of the imaginary comes undone, and the body takes on a new form, perhaps it is possible to invent a new imaginary, a new way of being, where the body's imaginary boundaries alter to incorporate a way of existing with alterations at the level of the organism.

## The Sinthomatic Body

It strikes me that there are some parallels between Artaud's project of inventing a new body through the deconstruction of language as an organising system and Lacan's later work on the sinthome and his emphasis on creativity and art as a modality of holding the subject together in a knotting of the three rings of the Real, the imaginary and the symbolic. In exploring this idea, I would like to take into account the potential for art per se to be an avenue of invention (a sinthomatic pathway) for subjects whose bodies fall outside conventional parameters or who have experienced the destruction of their original bodies through illness, disability, pain or other contingencies. This idea also has inherent limitations, as framing psychoanalysis as a somewhat clinical outcome for a subject who is not in analysis is not without conceptual and practical misalignments. However, Lacan's famous case study of Joyce in *Seminar XXIII*, in light of the sinthome, is of a subject who is not in psychoanalysis and, perhaps as a result of his art, did not need one.

Both Artaud and Lacan, and it is ironic to place both names in conjunction, given Lacan's damning assessment of Artaud, aimed for the Real, the realm of the unspeakable that is also the unnameable quality of corporeal affects and states, in their challenging of the limits of sense, signification, and finding avenues for the expression of the truth of being. Of course, Artaud seemed to believe in affects as an expression of truth much more strongly than Lacan but nonetheless, the path of invention towards a new signifier, as has been noted, was Lacan's later intention in *Seminars XXIII* and *XXIV*, and appears to have some common ground. This new signifier was to be a signifier devoid of sense, yet capable of resonating with the subject in a singular way. Is this also what Artaud was attempting with his sounds and bodily utterances, or was he more focused on creating a universal language in which the singularity of the Other (the desire of the Other) was effaced? Or could we even say that both positions can co-exist? I think it is probably the latter, as it is safe to say, as I already indicated in relation to sexuality, that he was traumatised by the lack in the Other; nonetheless, it is tempting to see this new signifier as the body without organs, not simply as a concept but lived as lalangue. We know Lacan was intent on moving away from the imaginary resonances of meaning, as is clear in his topological demonstrations and his attempt in *Seminar IX, Identification,* to identify a pure identification with the signifier that cannot be conceptualised or thought about in standard ways. In Lacan's later work, the symbolic becomes less the route for containing the Real and more a source of the Real—it has a parasitic dimension—we could say a tormenting dimension. In essence, the Real and jouissance come more to the fore as being the grounding of the subject. For Artaud, of course, his preoccupation was expressing the Real through artistic means or liberating the unconscious through affective experiences; for Lacan, it was through the process of analysis and putting into words, in the presence of another, the relation to the unconscious. There is a critical difference here in the position of how to live with the Real. For Artaud, the Real was managed through attempting to directly access the body, as if the affects of the body were somewhat superior to language. And yet this was not simply a personal project but an art form. The body itself is the canvas upon which a transmission of sorts could take place. So we have to consider Artaud's art in its entirety vis-à-vis the body, and not simply one concept, as being in the realm of the sinthome—as something that perhaps did not stabilise him but enabled him to live.

Lacan's seminar on Joyce explicitly deals with the question of how art functions as a fourth ring to stabilise a subject, or, in the case of Joyce, to prevent him from having a psychotic break. Lacan deduced that Joyce had a psychotic structure but that, through his writing and the invention of an almost new language or signification system, he was able to make a name for himself and create an ego structure in the place of the absence of a stable imaginary caused by the father's lack. It seems paradoxical to call the imaginary stable, given its inherent connotation of a precarious ego identification, but that depends on how we view identification—whether as that which alters or vacillates as a vacuous ego construction or as something deeply tied to the being of the subject. It would seem that identification is more in the latter category, and hence it is not so easy to switch or change our sense of self at the imaginary level. Indeed if we take Freud's viewpoint literally, that the ego is a bodily ego, this may involve changes or interventions directly at the level of the 'enjoying substance'. Certainly in his later years, the imaginary is assigned to the status of the body in the diagrams of the three registers. With the introduction of the Borromean chain, Lacan could illustrate the integration of the three registers as being of equal importance: if any one of them breaks or comes loose, the whole chain falls apart. As a result, it is important to note that in his later seminars, Lacan's position on the imaginary changes somewhat, and the imaginary is not simply a zone of misrecognition and illusory identity (relegated to that which isn't true for the subject) but grounds the subject more in a sense of bodily being than in ego identification as a mental construct. The stability of being consists, literally, in a tying together of the knot of the registers; without one of them in place, there is an unravelling, a rupture at the level of existence. In *Seminar XXIII*, while Lacan focuses specifically on Joyce's writing as providing the support of his ego and therefore of being, he also questions the role of art per se as providing the essential stability of the knot. In his words:

> How can art aim, in an expressly divinatory mode, to embody in its consistence, and equally in its ex-istence, the fourth essential term of the knot, how can it aim to render it as that such, to the point of approaching it as closely as possible?
>
> (Lacan, 1975–1976/2016, p. 10)

It would seem presumptive to state with any certainty that Artaud's art provided the fourth ring of the knot and served as a sinthome for his subjectivity, in particular, as there were other factors that regulated jouissance, such as opium, and the fact that his psychosis at times appeared to be florid. However, it is hard not to see Artaud's intent to create a universal language through performance as situated on the border between art and psychosis. In other words, perhaps it was an attempt to solve the disordered Other of the symbolic, a way of suturing the hole in meaning that, in Lacanian terms, results from the foreclosure of the name of the father that holds the symbolic together for the neurotic subject. Annie Rogers makes the point that psychotic subjects who invent a sinthome or create a new social link often don't need an analysis to manage their psychosis (2016, p. 198). We can ask, is what Artaud creates through his manifesto a social link, or does it work as a language? I think Murray makes a great point when she states:

> What Artaud communicates, or attempts to communicate, is his own corporeal experience; perhaps for this reason, his language can never be universal or transcendent in the way that he seeks. For him, his own experience is a reflection of universal truth, and his body becomes a microcosm of the external world. This does not take into account the possibility that the viewer, reader, or audience might not experience what he takes to be the 'direct' and 'immediate' physical response that he demands.
>
> (2014, p. 25)

Furthermore, as Rogers points out, the language the psychotic may invent is not interpretable outside its own code; the elements of the code only mean one thing: "The code reinstates the logic of the autonyms—it is complete, even as it emerges, and cannot be questioned" (2016, p. 85). Although this aside into the language of psychosis and the assumption of Artaud's psychic structure may seem to fall into the trap of interpreting art as biography, in doing so, something of the singularity of the body, in Artaud's case, is connected with a more universal extrapolation into the somatopsychic considerations of a theatre invented to 'speak' to the body. In other words, from Artaud's singular solution, we learn something of the limitations of transcending the body in general but also its potential transformation through art. We both are and have a body, and therefore, something is deeply rooted in our identification with the Real of the body, and something can be altered in our relationship to it at the level of the imaginary.

Added to this is, as Verhaeghe (2002) points out, we cannot save ourselves the trouble of analysis in working through the symbolic dimensions of our symptoms before we arrive at the Real kernel of jouissance beneath them, a kernel we must find a way of living with as something we identify with as a sinthome rather than believe in as a symptom. Despite this caveat, it might be more fruitful to think of Artaud's artistic endeavours, centred as they were on the body, as an attempt to plug the hole of the question of the body with an answer that had no meaning. The body cannot be known; like being, it can only be experienced—an experience that has a traumatic dimension.

## Narratives of Trauma

What can we learn about mind–body narratives from the Artaudian quest to make the body central in the pursuit of the inevitable evanescence of being? Also, in what way can we bring the concept of being as a question of the body into an understanding of bodily states of suffering, pain, and disability?

In many respects, Artaud's writing signals seminal texts in pain studies, such as Elaine Scarry's *The Body in Pain*, as he was intent on finding words for pain, even though, paradoxically, his writings express the difficulty of expressing it. Here is a direct correspondence with a theme in Beckett's work, as we saw in the previous chapter: the failure to express and the imperative to continue expressing that failure. Something is materialised, rendered visible through the inability to find the right or last words, the very imperfection of the symbolic. A sense of being debilitated from mental and physical suffering permeates his letters and poems, written through language cultivated to touch the depths of despair and to capture something of the gap inherent to thought and materiality. That Artaud himself had a nervous disability, as Martin Esslin calls it (1976, p. 17), is also a matter to note and up for discussion. In an essay on "The Liquidation of Opium" (1976, pp. 99–102), Artaud definitely identifies himself as aligned with those on the margins of society, those who are mad, ill, drug-addicted or disabled and expresses a view that the suffering involved in these situations is inexpressible in words but lends itself to depth and insight. His work certainly provides a platform for witnessing a subjective investigation and an attempt to express suffering in both body and mind. In the words of Sontag, "Nowhere in the entire history of writing in the first person is there as tireless and detailed a record of the microstructure of mental pain" (1976, p. xxi). Artaud would probably agree with this statement, given the emphasis on the superlatives of suffering in his writings and his self-professed debility. Of course it could be argued that these descriptions of physical and mental pain are not about disability per se and disability is not reducible to signifiers of suffering but is a social phenomenon caused by inequalities in the system and barriers to access. This, as we have seen, is the social model of disability. However, one of the most difficult things about bodily impairment and/or suffering is finding words to express it, particularly as it often falls into extreme categories where words or signifiers hardly exist to categorise the pain/impairment/limitation in question. Given that Artaud's life was marked by such intense suffering—including his subjection to electric shock treatment later in his life and his long-running opium addiction, which for many subjects could be completely consuming—the sheer volume of his artistic output is miraculous. His resilience and ascendance from the flames of his treatment in long-term confinement in the institution of Rodez to produce a further body of work that comprises the late Artaud, including his performance at Vieux-Colombier in 1947, is truly remarkable, a testament to a resilience of spirit and the reinventive arc of an artist resurrecting themselves from a breakdown of the self. As Stephen Barber (2003) poignantly recounts, Artaud was writing up to almost his final moments while he was dying of cancer.

Perhaps the answer to the dearth of engagement with Artaud in disability studies lies in the traumatic and excessive quality of his writings and theatre and the emphasis he places on pain and suffering. Also his status as a *poèt maudit* and his incarcerations in mental asylums may potentially deem him a figure that could bring a pathological evocation of the body into a field that resists medicalisation and psychiatric diagnoses of differential embodiment. However, Artaud's lifelong resistance to psychiatry and his insistence on the bodily basis of being provide fruitful avenues for critiquing normative conceptions of the body that deny the somatopsychic (body–mind) aspects of subjectivity. As is clear from his life and works, the trauma of the body can drive us to cultivate new ways of being in the world (the body as being) and new ways of relating to the body (as that which we have). While I do not want to be utopic here and argue that people with illness, pain or disabilities *should* find new ways of being through art or other sinthomatic modalities, I think that recognising the trauma at the core of not simply the body, but being, can be helpful in acknowledging that the suffering of the body is both structural and contingent to the human condition and that crises of identification are a natural response to alterations at the level of the body. Artaud is a bridge to considering this ontological trauma as central to the being of the subject and as something that can drive an interrogation of being. In his case, I also think we can see the limitations of aligning being with the body and the fact that while providing access to certain truths of being, manipulating the body as a corporeal substance does not provide a final solution to trauma. We can never be truly liberated from trauma as it is something structural, just like the Lacanian sexual non-rapport designates the incompleteness of the sexual relationship and the non-complementarity of the sexes as the central benchmark of the lack at the core of the subject's being. I argue perhaps contentiously that the trauma of the body can be more pressing for those who have suffered illness, disability or damage to the body in some way and that grappling with the question of being is one that surfaces for many people in these situations. So we could say that a contingent trauma, such as an accident or an illness, triggers the very trauma at the heart of the subject's constitution as an embodied being. While psychoanalysis may not often privilege the trauma associated with the contingent and accidental properties of the flesh, at the same time, as James Berger points out, the concept of trauma is an almost unspeakable issue within disability studies, arising potentially from a denial of loss and mourning inherent to the experience of impairment or physical difficulty (2004, p. 572).

I think this denial is a structural response to the 'not wanting to know' about the unconscious and its non-rapport with the body that permeates discourses, including ironically that of disability studies and psychoanalysis. As I quoted earlier in the book, psychoanalysis must be blown apart in order to expose its ableist prejudices and focus on the able productive subject of neo-liberal culture. The recognition that there is a structural component to trauma can help us understand the desire to cover it over with fantasies of a normal body that is impervious to lack and incoherence—as at any moment, due to contingencies of chance, we can be thrown into the pain of existing at the core of the fantasy.

Although I have been arguing for a theorisation of the body as traumatic for all human beings and that this structural dimension is evident in Artaud and Beckett's work, it is important that this does not become a narrative itself—a way of *not* saying something. In contemporary times, trauma has become a trope, a catch-all for complicated bodily or emotional states, a way of explaining mysterious phenomena, and thus another simplification for mind–body relations. The case I have been making is that this tendency to simplify is driven by an ontological trauma that drives the desire to know and indeed not know something about the body, leading to explanations that may miss the mark. To engage with the truth of the body is to wrestle with the very constituents of our existence—a being not fully expressible within language.

## References


Artaud, A. (1947). *To have done with the judgement of God*. https://surrealism-plays.com/Artaud.html.

Barber, S. (2003). *Blows and bombs. Antonin Artaud: The biography*. Creation books.

Berger, J. (2004). Trauma without disability, disability without trauma: A disciplinary divide. *JAC* Special Issue, Part 2: Trauma and Rhetoric, 24 (3), 563–582. Retrieved 5 September 2019.

Brenner, L. (2021). Is the autistic body a body without organs? In B. McLaughlin & E. Daffron (Eds.) *The body in theory: Essays after Lacan and Foucault*. pp. 42–56. McFarland & Company.

Deleuze, G., & Guattari, F. (1987). *A thousand plateaus: Capitalism and schizophrenia* (B. Massumi, Transl.). University of Minnesota Press.

Esslin, M. (1976). *Antonin Artaud: The man and his work*. Calder Publications.

ICLO (2025). *Flash cartel on Jacques-Alain Miller's text Lacanian biology and the event of the body*. Presentations given in Dublin.

Lacan, J. (2016). *The seminar of Jacques Lacan, Book XXIII: Le sinthome (1975–1976)* (J.-A. Miller, Ed.; L. Thurston, Transl.). Polity Press.

Miller, J.-A. (1999/2010). Lacanian biology and the event of the body (B. P. Fulks & J. Jauregui, Transl.). *Lacanian Ink*, 18, 7–29.

Murray, R. (2014). *Antonin Artaud: The scum of the soul*. Palgrave Macmillan.

Murphy, J. (2015). *Artaud's metamorphosis: From hieroglyphs to bodies without organs*.

Porcheret, B.(2020). *The bodily root of symptoms. Psychoanalysis Lacan Volume 1: Testimonies of the Pass*. Lacanian Circle of Australia uploads.

Rogers, A. (2016). *Incandescent alphabets. Psychosis and the enigma of language*. Karnac.

Ruti, M. (2012). *The singularity of being: Lacan and the immortal within*. Fordham University Press.

Shildrick, M. (2009). *Dangerous discourses of disability, subjectivity and sexuality*. London: Palgrave Macmillan.

Sontag, S. (1976). Introduction in *Selected writings* (S. Sontag, Ed., H. Weaver & D. E. Levine, Transl.). Farrar, Straus and Giroux.

Tubino, C. & Moschen, S. (2021). Scream scriptures in Antonin Artaud. *Psicologia USP*, 3, 1–11.

Verhaeghe, P. & Declercq, F. (2002). Lacan's analytical goal: "Le Sinthome" or the feminine way. In L. Thurston (ed.), *Essays on the final Lacan. Re-inventing the symptom*. New York: The Other Press, pp. 59–83.

# Conclusion

## The Enigma of the Body and the Truth of Being

This book posited that asking a question about the body opens onto the path of interrogating the truth of being and that through this question, we can deduce a split ontology inherent to Lacan's work, but also apparent in the comparative analysis of Artaud and Beckett, namely, the being of the subject and the being of the body. In the works of the authors, the body is not a known entity, something we can tie down with any certainty, but its representation and invocation speak to what cannot be known as a fissure in being. For all human subjects, the body has a traumatic component that is primarily ontological rather than contingent; it is built into the structure of being a speaking subject, but it is also particular to each subject's experience and the contingencies that may befall any of us. The paradox of embodiment is that we both are and have a body, and do not simply exist in a relation of having a body. The paradox of being and having a body can be traced through the comparisons and differences in the positioning/representation of the body in Beckett's and Artaud's works. I mean position both literally and figuratively; that is, how the actual body is presented, whether fragmented, disabled, entrapped, or traumatised, but I also include as position the relation we can deduce exists to the body, even when the body is not specifically present. This relationality to the body in its absence centres on the concept of the object a as that which is of the body but has no image, specific sound or representation. An encounter with the object a can be provoked through the senses but is not reducible to a physical sensation or material source. The function of the object a has a twofold dimension concerning both an inward perspective on the body as that which is a trace within the play/artwork and the outward reception of the artwork by the spectator. The corporeal impact of an encounter with desire, the potential of a performance to alter something within the spectator's psyche.

Recognising that being is not a monist concept and is related to the body has important implications for understanding the impact of contingent bodily traumas and the changes that can occur at the level of identification. There is potentially always a question of being at stake in bodily difference, accidental injury, pain, illness, and disability. Beckett and Artaud's work

DOI: 10.4324/9781003509622-14

situate important existential questions concerning our relation to the body: who are we when we are reduced to the ground zero of the body? How do we go on if the identifications we had previously, as grounded partly in the body image, come under attack and we lose any semblance of narcissistic mastery? What role is there for the imaginary in inventing new ways of being for the subject of the unconscious, which is also a subject of or to the body?

On the aesthetic level, within the authors' works, I also asked: if the body has a traumatic kernel, how can we read or account for this aspect of the body in theatre/literary works? And how will addressing this question help us elaborate on the mind–body narratives that perpetuate the idea of a whole or fragmented self? The idea of reading for trauma might seem oxymoronic, but if we expand the parameters of what reading implies, we can include our own perceptual/subjective response to a drama or performance, the ways in which our perspectives may be altered, and how this occurs. Fundamentally, this book has relied on the concept of the unconscious as that which disrupts any normative conception of the body–mind binary and as that which challenges conceptions of ableism and simplifications of mind–body relations that fall into the extremes of either/or thinking. Taking account of the unconscious enables new readings of the body that can challenge narratives within the socio-cultural domain, including both psychoanalysis and disability studies. The work of both authors relates uncomfortably to the field of disability studies—for Beckett, there is the fantasy of debility, a means to access the negativity of being, the body as a minus sign; for Artaud, pain and trauma is the path to experience a being of the body, a being that he wanted to transform or deform at the level of the imaginary and the Real. Artaud also wanted to transform the audience through the corporeal performance of the Theatre of Cruelty. In relation to reception and spectatorship, the unconscious was also a factor to consider in the staging of the body—how the unconscious may resonate through art to disrupt our identifications with our bodies. It is also inherent in the stylistic motifs of Beckett and Artaud, and in the relationship to the Other and the positioning relative to the object a, which differ between the two writers. In this positioning of the object a as a proxy of the Other, nuances concerning the question of the body are defined. This relationship can be configured within the terms of excess and lack, respectively. For Beckett, the place of the lost object a is exposed as lost—there is no other of the Other that will guarantee a final resolution to the question of what existence means or the cause of its absurdity. Godot will never come, but the absence of Godot marks a structural necessity of the human subject, in which the striving for completion and the arrival of a 'being to come' promise some sort of relief from the deformations and bodily hardships of existence.

In contrast, for Artaud, the mythical lost object a is sought through the modality of performance as a bodily presence or excess that could mitigate the split between the conscious and unconscious self, or between thought and body. Affect, pain and jouissance align and occupy a privileged position in Artaud's theoretical writings and in his vision for a body that could transcend the splitting of the signifier. Hence, presence, as it is imagined to be in the role of bodily emissions (voice, affect, noise), functions as a substitute for the irrecoverable absence of being that has resulted from the imposition of the signifier and the birth of the subject.

While Artaud attempts to provoke the truth of the unconscious through an embodiment of the theatrical spectacle and, by so doing, wake the spectator in body and nerve, liberating the conflictual forces within, Beckett's worlds are characterised by a quest to uncover the truth of being when everything is stripped away. However, this is a truth that cannot be said; it is not so much that there are 'truths' buried in the unconscious, but rather that the unconscious is the lining of truth that is not a concrete saying of truth—the truth can only be half said—but that which disrupts the rational, cognitive basis of knowledge.

For Artaud, his desire to liberate the unconscious through the spectacle's mechanisms and affective excess is a form of idealism, based on a model of the unconscious in which truth is buried and can be released. Artaud's innovations in form posed the question of being within bodily existence and the attempt to unveil a core nonmimetic self within the signifying structures of theatre. However, revealing a central core to the self is questionable. There is no authentic being we can reach through the sensations or affects of the body, as this will only be partial. Being is both a function of language and the body of jouissance.

While Artaud pursued the impossible quest of uncovering the truth of being through a modality of performance characterised by bodily affects, Beckett encapsulated this impossibility of encountering truth within the very structure of particular plays. For example, in *Waiting for Godot*, the dramatic action is circular, raising questions for the viewer about time, change, location, and meaning. There are allusions to a knowledge we (the spectator) do not have access to, nor do the characters. Who is this Godot? Will he ever arrive? Taking waiting at face value here is to diminish the effect that it is Godot's lack of arrival, the missed encounter, that points to something that has already happened, not that will or could happen in the future as waiting would imply. Godot does not appear as his nonappearance is structurally necessary to Vladimir and Estragon's existence, which is supported by waiting, as per the nature of existence. From this perspective, it is not so much who or what Godot symbolises (as meaning) that should be questioned but rather how this nonappearance or missed encounter of Godot structures the play (as non-meaning).

Thus, *Waiting for Godot* dramatises an existential question concerning cause and effect in relation to humanity. The structure of the play mirrors the topological space of the unconscious, with movement and repetitive action circling something that, at its core, does not make sense, yet is born of the 'sense' or meaning effects of the discourse of the Other. The continuation of the act of waiting in the play and the lack of an unveiling denouement symbolise that there is no single identifiable truth (meaning or signified) that can accurately account for our existence, nor are there truths buried in our unconscious that, if released, would bring us total freedom. Godot is a signifier without a stable signified, and applying any concrete symbolisation to this elusive meaning, such as a sign or referent to a version of God, misses the point of its sliding nature.

So if the play mirrors aspects of unconscious structure, can we say we can read the unconscious through the signifiers of performance? This is a difficult question that raises various caveats regarding the role of literature and artworks in psychoanalysis and the nature of spectatorship. If we can read for the unconscious, it implies that we can apply a methodology to extract a deeper, more hidden meaning from a text or performance. But can a text have an unconscious or can it resonate like the unconscious? We remember Lacan's dictum that the unconscious is structured like a language, not that it is a language. While works of art may be permeated by the unconscious, we cannot simply read them as if they were symbolic puzzles to be deciphered, as if the unconscious could be read through the artwork's signs and signifiers, certainly not in a mimetic sense. In short, we can say that although artworks cannot be reduced to representations of the unconscious, as the unconscious manifests through accident rather than by design and is somewhat outside of representation, they nevertheless form part of the bricolage of the Other discourse that forms the unconscious in the first place.

Therefore, examining artworks through the prism of Lacan's ideas does not entail reducing a dramatic literary work to a single interpretation of the unconscious but should open onto equivocation, and in this sense, it would be oversimplifying to reduce the 'meaning' of a text to a product of empiricism. Nonetheless, while attempting to create novel ways of looking at the body without succumbing to reductive interpretations, this has not been without a tension between giving 'examples' to support a view and trying to find an anchor within representation to pin down an abstract idea. However, binary methods of 'applying' psychoanalysis may be mitigated by viewing the nature of drama and literature as intrinsic to the structure of the unconscious rather than as imitation or mimesis. In other words, psychoanalysis, as theory and praxis, is already immanent to literature and drama, and vice versa. Indeed, as Lacan argues, "Poetic creations engender rather than reflect psychological creations" (Lacan, Session 13, 4 March 1958–1958, p. 248).

If poetic creations engender rather than reflect, they can directly influence the psychic and, indeed, physical life of the human being. Myth and the poetic structures of fiction are intrinsically linked to our psychological processes and poetry enters our imaginations and alters us as a result. Literature is both created from the subject and creative as the subject. It can formulate new metaphors to breach the realm of the unspeakable or the underrepresented. In this way, theatre/literature can inform some of the deficits in psychoanalysis—for example, the dearth of material on the subjectivity of non-normative embodiment. My hope is that the work of Artaud and Beckett has provided a platform for thinking through some of these issues and for showing how useful Lacanian analysis is in devising a model of the body that defies the dictates of capitalist, neoliberal, able-bodied ideology. This model can also be applied to psychoanalysis itself as a discourse that may, in part, deny bodily difference. Furthermore, extending the analysis to incorporate the question of being places emphasis on the importance of the body, whether in the Real, the Imaginary or the Symbolic as an entity that can leave us confronting the core questions of existence. We saw that, for Beckett, the question of being is formulated through the reduction of the body to ground zero, where an absence at the heart of being is made to appear as absence, and, as a consequence, we can deduce a relationship or positionality vis-à-vis the Other as lacking. Beckett's aesthetic of debility subtracts all possible avenues of escape for the being of the subject, bar the wanderings of imagination, and cultivates an experience of being marked by a minus sign. There is no substance to being as such, only an endless play on words and interrogation at the level of the I.

However, for Artaud, the body, as it manifests and as he appears to desire it to function, is the answer to the gap—the noncommensurability of meaning—that exists between the signifier and the signified. The body in its immediacy of sensation provides a canvas for a hieroglyphics of the self, where a seemingly universal meaning is transmitted through gestures and an extra-linguistic corporeal signification.

The relation to the object a situates the two authors with respect to both the body and being. Artaud attempts to embody the object a, whereas the object a is of the body but is no-body; it is an absence. It cannot be made to materialise but is the signifier of the lack in the other, the lack in ourselves. Beckett, in contrast, makes the object a present by cultivating its absence, thereby exhibiting a relation to the Other that lacks, that cannot hold the answer to being. By contrasting the two authors and their positions vis-à-vis the object a as an aesthetic style, we gain an understanding of the division of being as it concerns the body. Is this a kind of neo-Cartesian split of the subject of the unconscious into body and subject? Yes and no. I am proposing that being is not a unitary, essentialising concept, a stable backdrop of existence, and that we do experience a sense of divisiveness or alienation concerning our being, particularly when the body is ill or becomes more limited. This does not mean that the being of the subject and that of the body are not connected and that in Cartesian terms we are in two divisible parts communicating by the pineal gland. Rather, we cannot access full knowledge of either component of being due to a structural and causal rupture of sense that operates at both levels or aspects. Language is what gives birth to the subject of the unconscious, according to Lacan, but in doing so, it renders the body somewhat at odds with this subject. Language denotes a body but the body is not specifically just borne of language. The excess of the flesh exceeds the containing, nominating, creative function of language. At times of damage or injury to the body, the contingency of the flesh comes into our consciousness; we are aware of the vulnerability of our bodies—any physiological changes within this body deeply impact our sense of self. While this book frames the body as an Other, as an entity that is the source of trauma, both ontological and contingent, I hope it provides insight into why, sometimes, the best we can do is to live with this discordance and be content with a certain level of disharmony. We would do well to remember Beckett's words, " You're on Earth. There is no cure for that."

## References

Lacan, J. (1958–1959). *Desire and its interpretation: Book VI*. (C. Gallagher, Transl.). Unpublished.

# Index

For Product Safety Concerns and Information please contact our
EU representative GPSR@taylorandfrancis.com Taylor & Francis
Verlag GmbH, Kaufingerstraße 24, 80331 München, Germany